INSIGHT INTO ACUPUNCTURE AND SPIRITUAL HEALING

7 WAYS TO KEEP YOU HAPPY

DR WASFY YANNY

ISBN: 978-1-5151-6073-1

PUBLISHED BY:
10-10-10 PUBLISHING
MARKHAM, ON
CANADA

Contents

Foreword

Insight Into Acupuncture and Spiritual Healing drives you to health and happiness.

This book reveals the secret of looking after your body, mind and spirit. It gives you insight into the difference between eastern and western medicine.

It reveals to you a great potential of expanding your ability to be happy and on top of your health problems, lifted up by your spirit.

It gives you guidance about medical and spiritual healing which is beyond our limited understanding.

Raymond Aaron
New York Times Best-selling Author

Dedication

This book is dedicated to you, the reader of this book. The idea for writing this book came to me when I attended one of the workshops conducted by Raymond Aaron. I wondered why I was not where I wanted to be despite of my best effort. I had a moment of epiphany when I realised why. At this moment I had to write this book, not for me but for you.

This book is my way of acknowledging the importance of having a mentor and coach. As the desert fathers say if you are climbing a mountain for the first time you need to follow a known route; you also need a person who has been there before as a companion or guide. That is what the Greeks call geron or geronta, the Russians starets and the Egyptian abba, a title which in these languages means elder or old man.

The sheer amount of collective wisdom that I gained from interacting with my mentor and coach Raymond Aaron has changed my life for the better and I sincerely hope this book will change yours too.

Acknowledgements

I express my thanks to Lisa Browning for clarifying my thoughts on paper and editing the book. I also thank her for proofreading and eliminating embarrassing errors.

I thank my family who have coped and dealt with my eccentric personality during my time working on this book and supported my efforts without even knowing what I am writing about.

None of this would have been possible without my mentor and coach Raymond Aaron who supported me all the way along to live my dream. I wish to thank professor Brian Cooke for his kind offer to review the book.

Finally my first and last most humble gratitude to God who has given me the divine energy and the grace for allowing me this opportunity to make a difference in the lives of my fellow companions who came in contact with this book.

About The Author

I used to work as a consultant anaesthetist and during my work in pain clinics I learnt a few points of acupuncture for back pain and then I learnt from my colleagues how to stop nausea and vomiting after operations whilst no drugs can stop it for previous operations. That made me think that there is something different happening to patients. When I retired from the NHS I went for a Chinese course of acupuncture and TCM (Traditional Chinese Medicine) for six months, then another course for medical acupuncture. I started to treat patients, family members and friends with acupuncture and it was a great success.

I, therefore, decided to write a book about the experience and attended one of Raymond's seminars and have written this book in between your hands.

Patients' testimonials

I suffered from chronic low back pain for over 30 years, and had tried physiotherapy, osteopathy and various exercises to find long term relief over the years.

Once I had had a couple of sessions with Dr.Wasfy Yanny, I realised that acupuncture was giving me the kind of relief that I had been looking for.

Dr. Wasfy's professionalism and skill is of a very high standard, and his years as an NHS consultant in pain management give him the ideal background to perform the delicate techniques used in acupuncture.

I always felt at ease with him, and never suffered any discomfort during the treatments. I would recommend Dr. Wasfy to anyone who is looking for a holistic solution to their pain and physical discomforts.

Zane Wall
Engineering Manager
22/07/2015

I have suffered from migraines since a very early age and conventional (western) medicine was more of a band-aid than a cure. The first time I had acupuncture to treat my migraines was when I was 12 years old, which cured me until my mid twenties. I again lived with the odd migraine until they became more and more frequent.

In June 2011, I saw Dr Yanny for acupuncture and again, migraines are things of the past. I was treated with care and he explained about the process in great detail. The acupuncture was effective immediately and I have not suffered from migraine since that day.

I wish to extend my thanks to Dr Yanny for relieving me of this, at times, a crippling condition.

I would have no reservation in recommending his acupuncture treatment.

A Beggs
Banker
27/07/2015

This is my feedback after the acupuncture treatment that I received from Dr W Yanny.

I had acupuncture treatment for two different problems and I found it to be very successful and beneficial. The two problems are as follows:

1- I was very stressed and anxious 4 years ago and received acupuncture treatment from Dr Yanny, whicht has helped me to relax and I felt much better very fast after one treatment session.

2 - The second time I had acupuncture treatment for left shoulder pain 2 years ago and after two sessions I was free of pain up to this day.

I have found Dr Yanny to be very professional, with a good bedside manner. I would not hesitate to receive any further treatment and to recommend him to anyone.

L . Seifein
NHS Professional
18/06/2015

I have suffered from chronic gout in my right great toe for many years. Typically I get an episode every couple of months, with pain and swelling lasting from a couple of days up to a week, usually controlled with colchicine, an anti-inflammatory.

Whilst I was visiting London from overseas for my son's engagement, I had an acute severe attack, and was unable to walk or even put on my shoes. I did not have my medication with me so Dr Wasfy Yanny, a family friend, offered me a few sessions of acupuncture.

After Wasfy carefully listened to my concerns and examined the area, he started his first session. I followed up with 3 further sessions over my visit. After the first I experienced some relief, and with time and the additional sessions the pain was significantly alleviated. Thereafter I was able to enjoy the rest of my holiday, so I am extremely thankful to Wasfy for his treatment.

Since then I have never had a severe attack of gout. Any episodes I have now are usually mild and significantly less frequent. This has made a big difference to my quality of life since I enjoy long walks with my wife. I very much appreciate the treatment Wasfy gave me and would highly recommend acupuncture to others.

Raouf Awad
Accountant
24/07/2015

Note to the Reader

The information, including opinion and analysis, contained herein is based on the author's personal experiences and is not intended to provide professional advice.

The author and the publisher make no warranties, either expressed or implied, concerning the accuracy, applicability, effectiveness, reliability or suitability of the contents. If you wish to apply or follow the advice or recommendations mentioned herein, you take full responsibility for your actions. The author and publisher of this book shall in no event be held liable for any direct, indirect, incidental or consequential damages arising directly or indirectly from the use of any of the information contained in this book.

All content is for information only and is not warranted for content accuracy or any other implied or explicit purpose.

Chapter 1
Acupuncture

Acupuncture is a healthcare system based on ancient principles originating in China. It dates back over 2000 years and today is still commonly used, which is positive proof of its effectiveness.

It looks at pain and illness in a holistic way as indications that the body, mind and spirit are out of balance. The overall aim of the treatment is to restore the equilibrium.

Using subtle diagnostic techniques and focusing on an individual rather than their illness, ultra-fine needles are inserted into specific acupuncture points on the body. Stimulation of these points can correct imbalances in the flow of what the Chinese call Qi (pronounced chee) through channels commonly known as meridians to trigger the body's natural healing response.

Acupuncture has been found to deal successfully with a wide spectrum of both acute and chronic illnesses, from panic attacks to hot flushes, and asthma to joint pain.

Why does Acupuncture work?

This is a question that no-one can really answer but in my view, with a western medical background, Acupuncture treatment technique seems to balance the autonomic nervous system of the body, which regulates heartbeat, intestinal movements and sweating, to retain a healthy balance between relaxation, digestion and being prepared for action.

Studies have shown that Acupuncture stimulates the production of naturally occurring substances in the body. For example, an Acupuncture pain relief treatment helps the release of endorphins, which is medically recognised as the body's natural pain killer. According to evidence-based clinical research, traditional acupuncture safely treats a whole range of common health problems.

What are the most common ailments to be treated effectively?

Adverse reaction to radiotherapy and/or chemotherapy, allergic rhinitis, biliary colic, depression, dysentery, period pains, acute gastric pain, facial pain, headaches, high blood pressure, induction of labour, knee or shoulder pain, low back pain, morning sickness, nausea and vomiting, neck pain, post-operative pain, renal colic, rheumatoid arthritis, sciatica, sprains, stroke and tennis elbow.

What other ailments may also benefit from treatment?

Other ailments benefiting from acupuncture may include abdominal pain, bronchial asthma, cancer pain, competition stress syndrome, infertility, fibromyalgia, shingles, insomnia, labour pain, lactation deficiency, ringing of the ears, obesity, osteoarthritis, polycystic ovary syndrome, pre-menstrual syndrome, and spine pain.

Suffer from any of the above ailments and want to find out more?

Why not book yourself in for a free consultation session where we will use the latest diagnostic techniques and you can experience the effects for yourself of how Acupuncture could be the right form of complimentary medical treatment for you.

Dr Yanny is a Consultant Anaesthetist MBBCh, FFARCSI, who has a special interest in acupuncture, pain relief and regional analgesia.

He has a certificate of competence from the Healing and Acupuncture College Brighton and, is a member of the British Medical Acupuncture Society.

Please refer to the website
www.insightintoacupunctureandspiritualhealing.com

Electric Acupuncture

Electroacupuncture is an acupuncture technique that, comparatively speaking, has only recently been put into practice. It is believed by some scholars that electroacupuncture was used as long ago as the early 1800's by physicians in France and Italy. However, some believe it was discovered in the 1940's by Japanese scientists who were interested in making bone fractures heal quickly, whilst others claim that this technique was not fully developed until 1958 when acupuncturists in China started experimenting with it as a form of pain relief. Regardless of these claims, electroacupuncture is growing in popularity as a form of treatment, and is used by many practitioners of traditional Chinese medicine for a wide spectrum of conditions. In China they use it for anaesthesia for major operations such as thyroid and head and neck operations, but it only works for a small percentage of patients.

What is the difference between electroacupuncture and traditional acupuncture?

Electroacupuncture is quite similar to traditional acupuncture in that the same points are stimulated during treatment. As with traditional acupuncture, needles are inserted on specific points along the body. These needles are then attached to a device that generates continuous electric pulses using small clips. These devices adjust the frequency and intensity of the impulse being delivered, depending on the condition being treated. Electroacupuncture uses two needles at a time so that the impulses can pass from one needle to another. Several pairs of needles can be stimulated simultaneously, but no more than 30 minutes at a time.

Does electroacupuncture hurt?

Patients may experience a tingling sensation while being treated, which is most possibly due to the electric current. However, in the majority of cases the effect produced by the current is inconsequential , which means the tingling sensation might or might not be felt. Some minor bleeding or bruising may occur; this is a result of a needle hitting small blood vessels.

Are there any risks involved?

Electroacupuncture should not be used on patients with a history of seizures, epilepsy, heart disease or strokes, or on patients who have been fitted with a pacemaker. Also, it should not be used on a patient's head or throat, or directly over the heart. It is recommended that when needles are being connected to an electric current, the current should not travel along the midline of the body (an imaginary line running from the bridge of the nose to the belly button).

Before trying electroacupuncture, it is advised that patients discuss the potential risks and benefits with their practitioner.

One advantage of electroacupuncture is that a practitioner does not need to be as precise with the insertion of needles. The reason for this is because the current being delivered through the needle stimulates a larger area than the needle itself. A further advantage is that electroacupuncture can be performed without the use of needles. A similar technique called transcutaneous electric nerve stimulation (or TENS) uses electrodes that are taped to the surface of the skin instead of being inserted into the skin. A particular advantage of this procedure is that it can be used for people with a fear of needles or who suffer from a condition that prohibits them from being needled.

What conditions can electroacupuncture treat?

According to the principles of traditional Chinese medicine, an illness is caused when Qi does not flow properly throughout the body. Acupuncturists will determine whether Qi is weak, stagnant or out of balance, thus indicating the points requiring stimulation. Electroacupuncture is considered to be particularly successful for conditions where there is an accumulation of Qi, such as chronic pain syndromes, or in cases where the Qi is difficult to stimulate.

This technique has been studied in the United States for a variety of conditions and has been used effectively as a form of anaesthesia, a pain reliever for muscle spasms, and in treating neurological disorder. Further studies have examined the role of electroacupuncture when treating skin conditions such as acne, renal colic and acute nausea caused by cancer medications. There is evidence that electrical stimulation may enhance the rate of pain relief in certain conditions, e.g. back pain.

Meridian screening of acupuncture channels

Acugraph is another way of screening the energy channels if your practitioner uses Acugraph Digital Meridian Imaging system as part of an integrated approach to your healthcare.

What is an Acugraph?

The Acugraph Digital Meridian Imaging is a computerised tool used to analyse and document the energetic status of acupuncture meridians. Your practitioner will use the system in a short examination by touching a moistened probe to acupuncture points on your hands and feet.

What are Acupuncture Meridians?

Acupuncture meridians are invisible energy pathways in your body that have been used therapeutically for over 5000 years. These meridians conduct life force energy on Qi in and around all parts of the body. Blockage or interference in these meridian pathways can result in energetic imbalances that may contribute to negative health conditions. The primary goal of acupuncture treatment is to restore the energetic balance and proper energy flow of these meridians, thus allowing your body to function normally and return to health naturally.

How Can Acugraph Help Me?

The acugraph system allows your practitioner to measure and analyse the energy balance of acupuncture meridians. Armed with this information, your healthcare practitioner can make a better informed decision about your condition and provide the best possible treatment.

The Body Fields Energy Scanning

This is another way of screening the energy balances of your body and treating you accordingly.

A mother took her child who has cerebral palsy to a seminar for spiritual healers. Her child used to walk on his toes, heals up, and his left hand was closed and he could not open it. At the first session the practitioner put his hand around his body and in five minutes the child started to walk normally with his feet flat on the floor; he started to go upstairs normally instead of crawling on hands and legs. At the second session he had much improved hand function, he could hold a glass of water and drink and could give his mother a cuddle, something that he could not do before.

Traditional healing cannot explain that sort of rapid healing because it concentrates on body, mind and spirit. But reconnected healing can explain it.

If you put electromagnetic encephalogram around the head without penetrating the skin, it can read the brain activity and fields.

If we go back to Newton's clockwork theory he mentions that we have separate body, heart and mind. but that does not explain the healing.

We are not a chemical machine and our bodies react to medical drugs to a certain extent in acute disease but not for chronic conditions.

Today, with quantum physics and reduction mechanics, we can explain the molecules' collision of enzymes and hormones as a control system, but that does not explain what happened with the holistic theory for hundreds of years, there is a giant energy of the universe, there is a field information structured energy and the entire system talk to each other.

If somebody goes to a cathedral or a church and meditates, they can feel the effect of the quantum energy; so all matter is information structured energy.

In the nervous system not all the nerves, neurones are connected

How do they connect and communicate and coordinate?

They did a study on rats and trained them to cross a bridge and then they removed most of the rats' brains, and they still crossed the bridge. The conclusion was that our memory might not be in our brains.

A patient with irregular kidney function went to see a practitioner. He had a body scan and they found that his kidney was getting smaller in size.

He went to see a practitioner and was treated with information and energy transfer, Biophotoemission, and got cured. DNA, and genes cannot explain that.

Another story

A family with a history of cancer adopted a child from a family who had no history of cancer. When the child grew up in this family he acquired cancer.

Epigenetics, bleu prints and environment can affect the genes, so genetic fields are important.

All organs of the body have a magnetic fields, the strength of the electromagnetic fields differ enormously between organs. One field can organise the other body fields. The heart is the emperor and with its magnetic emission which is far more than any other organ in the body, it can affect the other electromagnetic fields of the body. It can be a coherent or incoherent pattern.

The heart gets the field of information then directs the brain and the body as to what to do.

There is neural information in the heart, and we are full of information in our bodies. In the ancient book of definitions (Neijing) in China it defines the heart as the ruler of the human body, the seat of consciousness and intelligence. It represents the body's imperial fire and the root of life.

Acupuncture is organised fields of information which can be interchangeable and it is possible to correct the distorted information.

It can cure cancer, fibromyalgia and allergy, and many other diseases.

This system is used in NES HEALTH for screening and treating patients. They invented ProVision so you can see the human body fields. With a single click of your miHealth or a special scanner, the software will immediately deliver a richly detailed overview, multiple screens and physiologically accurate graphics so you can see distortions in information, any energy blockages, and recommended nutrition for rebuilding the body. They use 4 R's: Reassess. Rejuvenate. Reimprint. and Rebuild for evaluation of total body wellness.

- Provision _ Reassess the energy and information of body fields
- miHealth device _Rejuvenate the body's energy blockages as seen by the Doctor's Show.
- Infoceuticals _ Reimprints the body back to its original and optimal blueprint using energy and information.
- NEStritionals _Rebuilds the biochemistry of the body nutritionally.

The Qi and the Main Organs

The Qi and its circulation

As you know the circulation in a human body, the left side of the heart pumps the oxygenated blood to aorta, arteries and capillaries and gives the tissues oxygen and nutrition then the deoxygenated blood is collected into the veins which goes back to the right side of the heart, the heart pumps it to the lungs to get oxygenated and goes back to the left side of the heart which pumps it to the tissues again, and so on.

In Chinese medicine the Qi is invisible and it circulates through the channels and nourishes your organs. These channels are sometimes called the meridians. The channels and organs are comparable to the landscape around you. Major motorways between cities and smaller roads to the towns, and other smaller side roads to more remote areas. So the network of the roads is similar to the network of the channels, cities and towns can be compared to the organs of the body. The channels are called or named after the organs they join up with. The channels can be blocked or deficient of Qi and the organ becomes starved of vital Qi. If this continues it will manifest as disease either physically, mentally or spiritually. Sometimes the problem is not in the channel but there is pollution or unrest in the towns and cities and the organs can be affected in the same way. There are 12 main channels and organs, and each channel is connected to the main organ it supplies and can connect/interconnect with other channels.

The main channels are the lungs, large intestine, stomach, spleen, heart, small intestine, bladder, kidney, pericardium, triple energises, gall bladder and liver. In addition to the main channels there are 8 extraordinary channels, 12 divergent channels, 15 connecting channels, 12 muscle channels and 12 cutaneous regions. The extraordinary channels help to regulate the Qi in your 12 main channels by acting as reservoirs and ensuring you have sufficient Qi circulating in your body. They also circulate your Jing, an essence around your body. The most important two channels in this group are called the Ren Mai and the Du Mai. The Ren Mai runs in front of the body and is called the sea of Yin channels. The Du Mai runs up the back of the body and is called the sea of Yang channels.

The acupuncture points are used in the treatment to either strengthen (stimulate) or, in other words, unblock the channel, or sedate which reduces the flow of the Qi through the channel.

Most acupuncture points lie along each of the main 12 channels, along with the Ren Mai and Du Mai. Points are best described as whirlpools or depressions where the flow of Qi is disrupted. There are more than 365 points on the body and each has its individual use. Some channels have more points than others. For example, the bladder channel has 67 points, whilst the heart and pericardium channels have 9 points each.

Some Interesting Points

Stomach 36

Some authors call it "chicken soup point of the body" because it is one of the most nourishing dishes in Chinese cuisine. That is because it is one of the most powerful points of the body. Some people call it "three miles leg" because it is used to strengthen a patient with depleted energy, and it is claimed that patients will be able to walk another three miles after treatment!

It has a beneficial affect on patients physically, mentally and spiritually.

There is a point just below Stomach 36 that becomes tender on pressure if the patient's appendix is inflamed.

Heart 7

The Spirit Gate is one of the most commonly used points on the heart channel. The name Spirit Gate gives us an insight into its ability to strongly affect the spirit of the heart. Also the name was given by many diarists? to the eyes as the practitioner can notice the vitality and brightness of the person's spirit from his eyes. It has a calming affect if the patient is feeling unsettled or agitated. One patient described the effect as a "whoosh of energy travelling straight up her arm, over her head and down her other arm" after which she felt completely at peace and did not want to move. She had felt the energy through its pathway resulting in wellbeing and relaxation.

GB 20 (Wind Pool)

One of the commonly used points to treat headaches.

There are too many causes of headaches and migraines and only the practitioner can decide which treatment you need. It is one of the points that treats headaches, especially tension headaches, and it has a magical affect on the headache, after which the patient often feels a dramatic difference from the first treatment and may not need to come back. It also eliminates wind, treats dry eyes, clears sense organs and activates the channels and alleviates pain.

What is Yin and Yang?

It is the concept of duality forming a whole. We encounter examples of Yin and Yang every day, for example – night (Yin) and day (Yang), female (Yin) and male (Yang). It represents the two opposite principals of life. Dark and light, hot and cold, passive and active, etc. Yin and Yang are not static or just two separate things. The nature of Yin Yang lies in interchange and interplay of the two components. It is the most known and documented concept used within Taoism.

The six evils, or pernicious influences, in Chinese Medicine are:

1. Wind

The word wind or "FENG" grasping the wind in Chinese is known as one of the six external causes of disease. It is associated with the five Chinese element theory (wood element), it can be of external or internal origin and is related to acupuncture point names e.g. fengchi (GB20), fengfu(GV16) and fengmen(BL12)

Wind in Chinese medicine can be used as the etiology or manifestation of disease.

Many diseases can be described in this category:

- Diseases involving excess movement of the body e.g. epilepsy (rare convulsions of the body) and Parkinson's disease.
- Diseases involving symptoms appearing in several parts of the body at different times e.g. early stages of rheumatism involving different joints.
- Diseases involving loss of movements such as stoke, paralyses, tetany and coma.
- Various pain, numbness and spastic symptoms, and sometimes referred to as bi symptoms e.g. headache, toothache, limb numbness, tendon spasms and arthritis.
- Diseases that are acute e,g, common cold, flu, nasal sinus infection, skin eruption, sore throat, cough and some eye disorders.
- Diseases that affect the surface of the body e.g. chronic eczema, leprosy, scrofula and hair loss.

In modern medicine, a number of causative factors have been identified for the "wind' disorders of concern, including infectious agents, neurological problems and auto immune diseases.

Despite progress in scientific analysis, the reason that a disease has manifested in any individual may be difficult to pin down. Furthermore the manifestation in different individuals may be markedly different. None of the modern explanations for the cause or manifestation of a disease or disorder inherently contradicts the traditional concept that they are caused by wind or somehow involve wind, and the explanation seems more detailed and up to date.

The availability of modern explanations raises the question of how useful the ancient terminology is when it comes to understanding the disease and deciding upon the method of treatment. Thus it is important to get a sense of how much reliance there is upon the basic concept of wind in Chinese medicine.

2. Cold

The cold pathogenic factor is considered a yin evil Qi. Its nature is to slow movements down, causing tightness, contraction, stagnation and impaired circulation. When it is external, pathogenic cold can cause skin problems, and it can affect muscles and the lungs. When it is internal, it can affect and cause impairment of the normal functions of the spleen, stomach and kidney.

Wind cold: In combination with the pathogenic factor, cold can attack the exterior of the body causing chills, lack of sweating, occipital headache, upper body aches, tight shoulders and neck, and a congested runny nose and clear secretions. The influence of the wind can cause the symptoms to appear suddenly. The treatment is to repel the wind and disperse the cold with worm diaphoretic herbs, acupuncture and moxibustion.

Obstruction Due to Cold

Traditionally called cold bi (blockage); patients feel body aches, joint pain which is relieved by warmth. The most common diagnosis in the western world is arthritis. The Chinese treatment is to increase the circulation, warm the acupuncture meridians though which the Qi and blood circulate by means moxibustion, acupuncture and herbs.

Cold attacking the spleen and stomach

This is caused by external factor which lead to digestive symptoms e.g. abdominal pain, clear vomit, watery diarrhoea, although it usually accompanies an externally contacted cold or stomach bacteria or virus and some people call it stomach "flu". This symptom can be caused by eating cold food e.g. ice cream.

Spleen Yang deficiency (deficiency of energy and heat in order to digest food)

Cold can severely impair the digestive system; it can manifest itself as watery stool with undigested food, cold extremities, oedema and slow pulse. Treatment aims to expel the cold pathogenic factor, then it tonifies the Yang aspect of spleen and kidney to bring about a long-term increase in your meridian energy, as the spleen is considered in TCM as the metabolic life gate fire.

Kidney Yang Deficiency

Kidneys in Chinese medicine are the source of Yang metabolic fire for the entire body. A deficiency in kidney Yan can make the individual especially prone to cold. The symptoms of kidney Yang deficiency are soreness or cold sensation in the knees and lumber region, aversion to cold, cold limbs, spiritual fatigue, difficulty in urination, enuresis, incontinence, declining libido or impotence in severe cases, female sterility and general oedema may also appear.

Cold can affect the liver meridian

The liver meridian passes through the genital area, and cold can manifest itself in this area causing testicular pain, retraction, hernia pain.

Moxibustion, acupuncture and herbs can relief the symptoms in a short time.

How do Chinese treat cold?

Basically they aim at increasing your immunity, and that will increase your body defences; prevention is better than a cure. This is done by diet, emotions and exercise.

Diet

Patients must first discover whether they have a hot, neutral or cold constitution. One way to do this is to take ginger. After eating a small amount of fresh ginger, do you experience excess internal fire, e.g. sweating, red swollen eyes, sore throat, thirst, dry mouth and constipation? If so, you lean toward a hot constitution (on the Yan side) and you should seek a cooling food such as watermelon, cucumber, soy beans to balance your energy. On the other hand if you tend to be on the neutral or cold constitution (Yin-leaning, which is characterised by cold limbs, low immunity, and an aversion to cold), you should search for warm or hot food e.g. chicken, meat, curry, garlic, wine etc. to move back to a balanced constitution. Traditional Chinese medicine discourages overeating. It believes that diet can restore balance inside your body, and improve your immune system, which acts as an auxiliary therapy with other treatments.

Emotions

TCM recognises seven emotions you keep in check. Those emotions are overjoy, anger, anxiety, overthinking, sadness, fear and fright. Optimism is the key to regulate emotions; TCM suggests brief centring/clear-the-mind techniques, or listening to calm inducing music.

Exercise

TSM recommends a slow, rhythmic, breath centric form of exercises incorporating all parts of the body, as opposed to the western approach which isolates body parts and muscle groups and is more strenuous.

3. Damp

In Chinese medicine dampness is the by-product of eating food that clogs the free energy flow in your body. A healthy diet might be completely different than what you think from the modern choices of what a dietitian recommends on television, magazines or diet books. It promotes diet which is based on energetic principles to encourage energy balance in your body, and clear your digestion problems, which leads to a healthy energetic body. As mentioned before, TCM believes that disease is the result of energy block or disturbance of the flow.

Damp Producing Foods

Popular food such as cheese, yogurt, white flower and sugar are all culprits in the formation of dampness. Dampness causes stagnation and manifests as mucus in the nose and lungs, digestive problems such as loose stools or constipation, obesity, or swollen joints. Some common diseases like allergies and arthritis are associated with dampness.

The Chinese believe that proper digestion is the cornerstone of Chinese medicine, and the foundation of good health.

When you eat some food it starts to get digested from your mouth, then goes to your stomach and small intestine, where most of it gets absorbed to supply the energy to your body, and the waste goes to the large intestine and gets expelled from the colon.

The Chinese diet includes all known spices, including ginger, which help digestion, and common foods e.g. pearled barley which helps with reducing the dampness. The aim is to balance the energy.

What foods do the Chinese recommend to reduce dampness?

Vegetables

Have you ever noticed the quantity of vegetables when you order a meal with vegetables in a Chinese restaurant? They serve you a heaped plate of lightly cooked vegetables. They believe vegetables play a major role in draining the dampness, and are full of life-giving nutrition.

Rice

Rice is a balanced food which is easily digested; it is the number one hypo-allergic food that is recommended for all patients who suffer from allergic conditions. Rice is a 'clean burning' food in Chinese medicine and it gently drains the dampness from the body.

Protein

The Chinese serve a small portion of animal protein or beans because they believe that it can be difficult to digest, hence the emphasis on 'small'. A serving size is usually 2-4 ounces, 3-4 times a week. Beans can be eaten more often as they absorb the dampness and provide the body with proteins and fibre.

You have noticed that they don't include cold raw food e.g salads, chilled food, iced drinks and frozen food. Also they do not include dairy products e.g. cheese, butter, milk on their menus. They believe that these products create dampness. The dairy products are building products and are suitable mainly for undernourished people. In a culture concerned about calcium and in the western world people depend on dairy products to provide them with calcium. All calcium needs can be met with several servings of vegetables per day, adding small servings of salmon almonds and leafy greens. to your diet each week.

No Cold Raw Food

This includes salads, chilled food, iced drinks and frozen food, because in TCM they believe these cold foods are difficult to digest, and in order for your body to digest, process and extract the essence from the food it has to be warm. Heating food inside your body strains your energy resources, weakening your energy system over time.

No Dairy or Dairy Products

The Chinese menu does not include milk, cheese and butter. They believe that the energetic nature of dairy is cold and hinders digestion. So they recommend it only for undernourished people and babies. Calcium can be replaced by eating almonds, salmon, leafy greens and broccoli; other minerals are equally important in the formation of strong bones.

Sugar

Concentrated sweets like soda, candy, sweetened yogurt and energy bars quickly create damp and are greatly overeaten in the western world.

The Chinese food is primarily sweet, and sweet is considered nourishing.

By sweet, the Chinese means rice, animal proteins and vegetables.

Sugar impairs the body's ability to transform food, and incompletely transformed food becomes dampness.

4. Heat

Associated with the heart, summer time, fire element, Yan evil. It dries fluids which can lead to Yin Xu, heat rises and appears on the face, eyes and nose, and causes redness. The more red the more heat. When it affects you it easily produces winds. It speeds things up, which leads to agitation, restlessness and can cause bleeding. It can affect the skin with red, itchy and painful rashes.

It can cause too many syndromes: wind heat, damp heat, excess fire.

Symptoms of fire

Lung fire
Can be a loud, forceful cough with blood, the sputum turns to yellow, green or brown. The skin can become full of a red painful rash.

Stomach fire
Buning ulcer, heart burn; it can cause toothache as it lies on the stomach channel, or frontal headache.

Heart fire
Strong anxiety, restlessness, insomnia and mania.

Liver fire
Anger, shingles in the intercostal area and burning pain in the genital area.

Large intestine fire
Dysentery, toothache (Channel pain) which is more tan than the kidney fire, long term alcohol or drug abuse, bone infection and meningitis which can affect the bone marrow.

Deficient fire
Yin Xu, Yang Kan, heat is deep in the body. Ying (nutritive Qi) level is a pattern of mixed Xu (deficiency) and excess.

Treatment must include quelling the fire as well as nourishing the Yin.

Smouldering heat especially at night, low grade rashes, severe restlessness, slight bleeding, tongue colour is scarlet and the pulse is thready and rapid.

5. Summer heat

Characterised by high fever, restlessness, thirst with strong desire to drink, can go up and affect the head, dizziness, blurred vision, headache, constipation, small amount of dark yellow urine, coma, Yin collapse, profuse sweating, dry red tongue, surging pulse (flooding-strong, big waves).

If it is combined with dampness it results in nausea, vomiting, diarrhea, poor appetite and fatigue, phlegm can rise to head, dizziness, heavy head, foggy thinking, suffocating or tightness feeling in the chest, profuse sweating not as much as summer heat without dampness.

6. Dryness

It is associated with the Lung, Autumn, Metal Element and Yang evil. If it is exterior in origin it is easily damages the body fluids, the effect of which is dry skin, dry hair, dry eyes, dry lips, dry throat or low grade sore throat, dry stools, scant urine and thirst. It can easily damage the lungs; could be from dry climate or smoking, and could result in dry cough and dry phlegm (thick, sticky and hard to expel).

Symptoms of dryness

Warm dryness
Characterised by fever, headache, thirst, dry mouth, dry nasal passages, dry cough and phlegm, red tongue with thin or no coat and rapid pulse. It can be treated by acupuncture and drinking plenty of fluids and not eating unless you are hungry. If it is chronic it is important to tonify the Yin.

Cool Dryness (e.g. dried out from air conditioning)
Characterised by dry phlegm, sensitivity to cold, chills, mild fever, headache, dry cough, dry mouth, dry nasal passages with stuffiness, tongue is thin and white, tight slow pulse. It can be treated as wind cold.

Chapter 2
Medical Acupuncture

How is it Different from Chinese Acupuncture?

The main difference is that the ancient beliefs of Yin Yang and the energy of Qi is substituted for a combined knowledge of physiology, pathology, anatomy and the common principles of evidence-based medicine. Medical Acupuncture is practiced by healthcare practitioners and is generally regarded as part of conventional medicine. The National Institute for Health and Care Excellence (NICE) recommends the use of acupuncture specifically for lower back pain.

What can you Expect from a Medical Acupuncture Appointment?

You will be referred to a medical acupuncture trained doctor who will diagnose you using Western medical methods. He or she will ask about your habits, lifestyle and medical history. Your blood pressure is usually measured and treatment administered once or more a week for a maximum of six weeks.

Is it Safe and Hygienic?

Yes. Only sterile, single use disposable needles will be used. He or she will decide to use electric acupuncture or not.

Does it Hurt?

You might feel a sharp sting or feel something like scratch or feel nothing. Most people feel very little.

What You Need to Tell Your Doctor Before a Medical Acupuncture Appointment

1. If you have ever fainted, had a fit or experienced a "funny turn".
2. If you have a bleeding disorder, e.g. haemophilia
3. If you have damaged heart valves, suffered from rheumatic fever or are at particular risk of infection.
4. If you have a pacemaker or any implants of elective nature.
5. If you are on anti-coagulants, e.g. Warfarin, Aspirin, Plavix, or any other medication.

Side Effects of Medical Acupuncture

Do not drive immediately after your appointment as you may feel drowsy or sedated.

Some people do faint during treatment (very rare).

There is a slight possibility of minor bleeding or bruising after the insertion of acupuncture needles.

Does it Work?

There are a lot of studies looking into the validity and benefits of acupuncture as an accepted form of medical practice. One study says that it seems acupuncture only appears to work by inducing a placebo effect. A placebo effect is what happens when a person believes they have been treated. Recovery and pain relief is thought to happen as a result of this sense of belief and expectation.

However, there is a study published in the NeuroImage Journal that claims to have found scientific evidence that acupuncture does, in fact, have a direct effect on the body. In another study researchers in Southampton University and University College, London, used PET scans to monitor the brains of fourteen participants during three separate interventions.

In the first intervention the participants were prodded lightly with blunt needles and informed that the needles would not penetrate the skin or hold any therapeutic value.

During the second intervention the participants were prodded with specially designed false needles that telescoped in on themselves upon contact with the skin in the same way that a stage dagger does. However, the patients were told that the needle would penetrate the skin and the treatment would hold therapeutic value.

The third intervention involved the insertion of real acupuncture needles into traditional acupuncture points. The results of the PET scan showed significant differences in the brain activity during each separate intervention. During the first intervention when participants knew they were not having needles inserted in them, the area of the brain associated with the sensation of touch became active.

During the second intervention when the participants thought they were having needles inserted in them, the area associated with pain relief became active.

During the third intervention when the participants were having needles inserted in them, the area associated with pain relief became active but, interestingly so did another part. The region of the brain thought to be involved in the judgement of pain is known as the insular.

These results do suggest that Medical Acupuncture can affect the body beyond the placebo effect.

Acupuncture Within Physiotherapy

More and more physiotherapists are integrating medical acupuncture into plans to manage the relief of pain and inflammation. Physiotherapists work on the premise that acupuncture can help to relieve pain by stimulating the brain and nervous system to produce naturally occurring chemicals which include beta endorphins and naturally occurring peptides.

Acupuncture for Palliative Care

Medical Acupuncture is increasingly being used in conjunction with conventional medicine as part of a Palliative Care Plan. The techniques will be more gentle and soft but certainly can help, and the benefits can be numerous for symptoms such as acute and chronic pain, nausea and vomiting, xerostomia, vasomotor symptoms, fatigue and dyspnea. Many symptoms occur in cancer patients well after their initial treatment, which may include surgery, chemotherapy and radiotherapy. Patients might be helped with their psychological and physical challenges. Usually pain is treated first and then non-pain symptoms like hot flushes and dyspepsia. Radiation can cause bowel and bladder problems. Usually the analgesic effect of acupuncture wears off more quickly towards the end of life in contrast to other symptoms like hot flushes and dyspepsia.

Seven key steps towards a balanced healthy lifestyle.

1. Be satisfied with what you have but be ambitious.

2. Be happy even if you have any pain in your life.

3. If you have an ailment or disease do not wait too long to see a doctor, acupuncturist or spiritual adviser.

4. Exercise, as you need a healthy body.

5. Look after your soul.

6. Look after your spirit.

7. Have a healthy lifestyle.

Chapter 3
Be satisfied with what you have and be ambitious

What makes us unhappy in a world of greed?

1. You want more and more, and compare yourself with others. "Why don't I have what he has?"

2. All or nothing. If it is not black it is white, or if it is not perfect it is not good. Either you are for me or you are against me. If you do not do that you certainly do not love me.

3. Why is always happening to me, as some people exaggerate what is happening in their life. Others say, I am not going to like this as they jump to negative conclusions.

4. I feel it so it must be true. You might feel helpless in the face of a problem and conclude that there is not a solution. If you label yourself as a failure you talk yourself into being one. You cannot judge yourself or others on the basis of one incident. If you fail one exam there is always another chance.

5. I should do this, you should do that. Some people feel they should clean a room in a house or tidy the garden and this feeling feels like an obligation. With this same feeling they also want to boss the people around them. This person looks scruffy; he should look after himself and always look like a smart man. You should judge yourself before they judge you.

6. If things go wrong it is my mistake. You should take responsibility for your own decisions and mistakes happen to everybody. Wrongly taking responsibility for what everybody else does is not.

Emotion can be harmful

These harmful emotions can poison your mind in the same way cyanide can harm our bodies. In extreme situations it can kill you or lead to serious illnesses, e.g. heart attack.

Examples of these emotions include anger, hate, blame, cynicism, hostility, jealousy, revenge, resentment, suspicion and indifference.

Ambition

An ambitious person is a person who wants to attain a high status or position in life. For instance, somebody working in a company as a waiter has ambitions to become the manager or the owner of the company. Reigning in ambition is a term used when someone has goals or dreams that are too aggressive or above their capacity to achieve. Ambitious people are not dreamers; they really do intend to get to the top, and are often prepared to be ruthless to get there.

> *"Intelligence without ambition is like a bird without wings."*
> -- Salvador Dali

Every way of a man is right in his own eyes, but the Lord judges the heart. We live in a world where we can describe this generation as contradictory from the deliberate attempt of the media to manipulate and confuse the reality, to exaltation of the paradoxyms and irrational emotions in religion. We have succumbed to the universal tragedy of monotonous moral inconsistency. So we hear "I'm sick and tired of". Our world is so devoid of meaning, sanctity, trust, hope and the prevailing spirit of the age, so the reply to issues of the most importance is, "so what?" or "I don't care."

We have become abused and devalued by broken promises and nothing gains our interest any more. So some people fantasise after the abnormal, the unreal and the perverse to find relief.

So is there contradiction between being satisfied and your ambitions?

The law of non-contradiction is undeniable. A lot of people have their own ideas and thoughts and try to say other people cannot know anything. Our ideas and actions are relative to concrete truth. To see it differently, the law of non-contradiction cannot be denied without affirming and believing it. The law says two opposite things cannot be true at the same time in the same sense. An example of this is you either exist at the moment you read this or you do not. Your actions speak louder than words no matter how loud, sophisticated or enthusiastic you may profess things.

When the mouth admits the heart: a wilful denial is immoral, as such theories leave their believers confused and bemused in areas of knowledge and morals. The philosophy of meaninglessness was essentially an instrument of liberation. For example, we objected to the morality because it interfered with our sexual freedom, or we objected to our political and economic system because it is unjust. The problem is that sometimes we say we don't know because we don't want to know; it is our will that decides. Those who decide or detect no meaning in the world generally do so because for one reason or another it suits their wishes that the world is meaningless.

Faithful Truth Of Investigation

It is only for those who seek the truth that life is worth living. We have talked about the law of non-contradiction. Therefore, we must apply it to everything we investigate. If something is proved to be true then the opposite is false. If there is God then atheism is false. If Jesus has risen by his own divine power then the doubters are wrong. If this proves to be the only way then all the others are wrong. If you let any known truth remain uncommitted in your life, then you will be ultimately deceived. It is only intellectual gluttony to reach for more truth when you refuse to be faithful to and thankful for what you already have. The object of the truth is to be lived. If you fail to do so you have missed the key ingredient to life. If we take the time to honestly and reverently seek the truth (without getting impatient and prejudiced) we will find it. The problem is that we will never see it properly if we seek it solely for ourselves. This is a great mystery, which is why the truth is so obscure and foreign to so many, especially amongst the educated and the half-educated. They fail to see that fundamental truth comes only with a benevolent heart. They think it comes from the most developed reasons and facts. They thought it and never found it because they stumbled over the stumbling stone of sin and they did not understand "it is better to give than to receive". Sometimes you need to cancel your thinking to believe in God or in another way believe by your heart. The most important questions in life, origin, meaning, morality and destiny.

Chapter 4
Be happy even if you have pain in your life

Being happy doesn't mean that everything is perfect. It just means that you have decided to look beyond the imperfections.

Even though I do not care about oil-based raincoats, I listened to a 15 minute talk on the subject one wet, rainy morning.

There is a small guy, who wears a colourful button-down shirt and odd-looking hat who makes my day in the mornings. He works at the café where I buy my coffee and he always appears happy. At first I thought he was putting on a pleasant smile to make the best of a bad situation. I thought, surely he can't possibly enjoy working in a café. Then I realised I was missing the main part of his appeal: he does enjoy his job, and the reason he always looks so happy is because he is!

Life doesn't always appear how I want it to. A lot of my time is spent in my living room writing alone when I would prefer to work in a beachside office shared with good friends. I drive an old car when I would prefer a newer model that doesn't have roll-up windows or a cassette player. I know that the world won't change despite having more money, a better job or a shiny new car. The wrapping paper may be different but the gift remains the same.

The way I feel about myself, how I approach new people and experiences, whether I smile just because it feels good – none of these depend on my life situation. I suspect the guy in the café knows this, too.

1. If you are always looking towards tomorrow to achieve happiness, the odds are you will continue to do the same when you have attained your dream. It may sound odd, but the ability to appreciate what you have in front of you has nothing to do with what you actually have. It's more about how you measure the positive things in your life at any one time. Practice wanting what you have and it will feel even sweeter when you eventually have what you want.

2. Dr Dacher Keltner of the University of California claims she can predict a person's future by the strength of their smile. Researchers examined Yearbook photos of 111 female students taken between 1958 and 1960. Subsequent tests showed that the women who expressed more positive emotion in those photos became more mentally focused, had more successful marriages and enjoyed a greater sense of well-being.

   "While positive emotion tends to broaden thought, negative emotion tends to narrow it and hold back development of brain and body. The findings of Dr Keltner and his colleagues, published in the Journal of Personality and Social Psychology, are among the first to show that differences in the extent to which people express emotion my be stable throughout their lives and dictate personal and social success."

3. Tuning into joy can improve your health, something that affords you many possibilities in life. This is something that most people take for granted until it is compromised.
   Christopher Peterson, Ph.D of the University of Michigan, has studied optimism's link to health over a period of twenty years. This study shows that optimistic people have a stronger immune system than their negative counterparts. This may be due to their tendency to take better care of themselves.

Choose to be happy now and you will enjoy more days of good health.

4. Once you get everything you want, you will still experience life's highs and lows. If you do not learn to enjoy the little things in life your well-being will parallel your life's circumstances. For instance, when something goes wrong you will feel extremely unhappy (as opposed to disappointed but determined to make the best of a bad situation). Think positively about what fills you with joy – spending time with your pets, running along a beach, listening to the sound of rain falling. Focus on these things now and let them brighten up your day. By doing this, you will have a variety of simple pleasures to help you regardless of what changes occur.

5. I used to be obsessed with being perfect. If I wasn't the best at something, I was unable to sleep at night. Becoming great never actually felt as good as I had imagined because there seemed to be room to be even better. I was always dissatisfied and disappointed in myself.
    I now view things as an opportunity to get better from one day to the next. It is much more gratifying to set and meet an attainable goal, such as focusing better and maybe writing an extra article tomorrow, than it is to obsess about perfection and feeling stressful because I am not a world-famous author.
    By focusing on small improvements and goals, you will move yourself naturally towards your bigger dreams and respect the way in which you are doing things.

6. You may think life needs to change dramatically before you can be the person you strive to be. You cannot give unless you make more money, or you are unable to be adventurous until you have sold your house. The truth is, of course, that

you can be those things at any point in time. So what if you don't have money to share. Be generous with your compassion, and listen to friends when they share their problems. So what if you can't sell your house. Try new things to bring adventure into your life and introduce yourself to new people. You never know when your "nows" will run out so ask yourself the question, "How can I be the person I want to be at this moment?"

7. Though we all have different lists of dreams and goals, for the majority of us this is at the forefront: the possibility of living a meaningful life that will affect other people for the better. Happiness is a moment-to-moment choice, a choice many of us find hard to make. Other people will notice when you have made this choice and this could motivate them to do the same. As indicated by this research, such motivation has a significant impact on their health and future happiness.

I know this isn't your usual "reasons to be happy" post. It didn't begin or end with "count your blessings", nor did I delve into your relationships or good fortune. There is a very good reason for this. I don't think happiness is primarily about what you have as this changes; your "blessings" evolve. Happiness is all about how you interpret what's in front of you and how proud you feel about the way you have led your life. This includes being willing to enjoy life's simple pleasures even when things may not appear perfect.

Although I have not always put this into practice, today I choose to focus on the good – both in myself and the world – and to feel happy now. How will you tune into happiness today?

Chapter 5
If you have an ailment or a disease do not wait too long to see a doctor, acupuncturist or spiritual healer

For example, if you have abdominal colic it could be several things; it could be sharp, stabbing, dull ache or colicy. It could be a simple food problem, bacterial, viral causes, or it could be serious, e.g. myocardial infarction, diabetic ketoacidosis, lower lobe pneumonia, sickle cell disease, high blood calcium, familial mediterranean fever, irritable bowel syndrome, urinary tract infection, gynaecological problems from pre-menstrual pain, to endometriosis on ovulation, or pelvic inflammatory disease. It could be a gall bladder problem, gastric or duodenal ulcers. It could even be something serious such as dissecting aortic aneurism, cancer or a volvulus. There are so many causes of abdominal pain and these are just a few of them. In addition, it can also be psychological. So do not wait too long before you see your own doctor.

You have read about what acupuncture can treat or improve, although every day new illnesses are added to the list which can be treated by acupuncture together with new techniques for the diagnoses and location of the needle points.

The Chinese also treat the evil spirit by acupuncture; they call it the Dragon. They wear white coats and open the windows to let the dragon out. With Good Spirit the complexion has lustre, the eyes have lustre and brightness, the mind is clear and alert and their respiration is even. The opposite is true with an evil spirit.

On the other hand, with an evil spirit there might be one or more of these symptoms.

1. Sudden drug or alcohol abuse. Suddenly drinking or craving alcohol more so than usual is a sign that you may have company.

2. Unusual behaviour from a young age. You may have picked up a wandering soul early in your life and you have endured abuse, serious illness and it might still be with you.

3. Excessive emotional stress breaks down your spiritual defences and opens you up to strange energy.

4. Acute unexplained bouts of depression. If you cannot explain this source it is possible you might be carrying a heavy unseen spirit.

5. Hearing voices in your head. Negative messages could be a sign of a spiritual hitchhiker with you or that you are hosting a party with uninvited, invisible guests. It is possible for problematic or other dimensional energies to plant ideas in your head and manipulate you behaviour for their benefit.

6. Reading this information and having a strong critical reaction to it. If you have a dark energy with you they will do anything to convince you to ignore advice that would lead to identifying them and being escorted away. You might experience subconscious fear which could be the reaction of unseen entities and since you are so used to it you believe it to be your own.

The good news is that it is rare, even for the darkest of other dimensional energy, to cause harm to you if you are aware of it and take measures to protect yourself from it.

Chapter 5
Exercise

If you wish to feel better, have more energy, suffer less coronary heart disease, boost your mood and improve your sex life, look no further than exercise.

Exertion controls weight

It can prevent excess weight gain and help maintain weight loss. With regular exercise you will burn more calories and, provided you do not eat compensatory snacks or consume high calorie drinks, you will lose weight. Some researchers claim you can lose more weight by dropping a meal a day rather than exercising for long periods of time.

Exercise can prevent health conditions and disease

If you worry about having a heart attack or high blood pressure, exercise can lower your blood pressure and can boost high density lipo proteins (HDL), good cholesterol and decreased unhealthy tri-glycerides. Regular exercise can prevent a lot of health problems, e.g. stroke, peripheral vascular diseases, high blood pressure, Type 2 diabetes, depression, arthritis and falls.

Exercise improves the mood

It can give you an emotional lift or, if you need to "let off steam" after a stressful day, a workout at a gym or a brisk 20-30 minute walk can help. Remember to consult your doctor if you suffer from chronic health problems.

Physical exercise stimulates various brain chemicals that make you feel happier, relaxed and can relieve or reduce pain. You will also feel better about your appearance and yourself following regular exercise.

Exercise boosts energy

If you worry about the amount of housework to be done, or a long shopping list, regular physical exercise can boost your energy and endurance. It increases the delivery of oxygen and nutrients to your tissues and improves the efficiency of the cardio vascular system; it also improves heart and lung efficiency.

Exercise improves your sex life

If you feel too tired or out of shape to enjoy physical intimacy, regular exercise will make you feel better, give you more energy and may have a positive effect on your sex life as it enhances a woman's arousal and reduces erectile dysfunction for men.

Exercise promotes better sleep

Regular physical exercise can help you to fall asleep faster and deepen your sleep, but do not exercise just before going to bed as you might be too energised to fall asleep!

Exercise can be fun

It gives you a chance to have fun, unwind, enjoy the outdoors, engage in activity that makes you happy.

Some authors think that running should be viewed as a wonder drug analogous to penicillin, morphine and the tricyclics.

Physical activity is positively associated with good mental health, especially a positive mood, general wellbeing and less anxiety and depression. Contrary to everything you may believe, exercise makes you happy and is fun, and there is no surer way to boost your mood, both immediately and in the long term. Scientists can measure these things as they have found that the level of endorphins, Phenylethylamine and your epinephrine shoots up with exercise; they may call them happy chemicals. Hormones and their actions in your body are so complicated. For example, more adrenaline is released if you are stressed and raises your blood pressure, which is bad for you. However, when you are happy, phenylethylamine is present and you feel great, and if dopamine is also present you will feel euphoric. So it is not only one hormone but usually a cocktail of hormones that have an enduring affect and helps you smile through life's little crises. If exercise bothers you, you could call it "optimising your physicality." It is not just a matter of producing happiness chemicals or strengthening your heart and lung systems and various muscles; it is also about improving the function of every part of your body. It is about feeling vital, animated and alive, feeling and being healthy; that will make you feel happy.

It is not only good for young people, but for all ages. It is the fundamental cause of happiness, particularly for older people where health equals happiness and happiness equals health. People who exercise a little every week enjoy two extra years of life compared to people who do nothing. People who exercise moderately enjoy almost four years extra, and people who exercise on a regular basis gain as much as ten years!

So what are you waiting for? Enjoying your body does not have to be painful or boring. Think about the gym, dancing, aerobics, skiing, volleyball on the beach, or football. Do whatever you fancy doing to keep fit.

Join the 20% and be happier, sleep better, have more energy, look and feel better, think more clearly, enjoy self-esteem, handle stress easier, reduce heart disease/heart attacks, increase your HDL levels "good" cholesterol, lower your blood pressure, increase your bone density, boost your immune system, enhance your sexual function and increase your life expectancy.

Consult your doctor if you have any medical conditions that can be adversely affected by exercise, e.g. heart disease, lung disease, diabetes, chest pain when exercising or difficulty with breathing during mild exertion.

Exercise is a Depression Buster

As exercise is so good in improving the mood it is now used as a standard treatment of depression. The National Institute for Clinical Excellence (NICE) recommends exercise and psychotherapy rather than anti-depressants as first line treatments for mild depression, but it can benefit all types of depression. As it is beneficial for depression you can get rid of the drugs and their side effects if your doctor allows you to do so.

The Happy Chemicals

Why does exercise make you feel good? It is hard to understand all the mechanisms that lead to the production of all these chemicals. Our ancestors had to be capable of vigorous activity if they were to eat. They were slim, strong and lived longer. These chemicals relieved their muscle pain.

Endorphins: this word means endogenous morphines, that is to say morphine-like substances produced naturally by our body. It relieves pain and promotes happiness. It is one of the ingredients of "runners high".

Phenylethylamine (PEA): It is also found in chocolate and some fizzy drinks. It is a powerful anti-depressant, and its level increases significantly following exercise.

Noradrenaline: When generated by exercise it tends to make you feel happy, positive, confident and creative.

Serotonin: This is a neuro-transmitter for happiness and scientists think exercise elevates its level in the brain.

Exercise lowers the level of cortisol, a stress hormone which is linked with low mood.

Exercise increases body core temperature, relaxes the muscles, increases blood flow of body organs, including the brain, and induces a feeling of tranquility.

Exercise increases the blood flow of the right side of the brain ("reactive thought") and decreases the flow to the left side of the brain ("logical thought"). This is why solutions to intractable problems may be found during exercise.

How Much Exercise do I Have To Do?

The surprise is, you do not have to do a lot of exercise.

Endorphines increase five times after 12 months of vigorous exercise.

Phenylethylamine (PEA) running at 70% of the maximum heart rate for 30 minutes increases phenyl acetic acid in the urine by 77% which is a metabolic of PEA.

Nor-adrenaline increases up to ten times following eight minutes of vigorous exercise.

1. Calculate your maximum heart rate (MHR)

You can work this out at a fitness laboratory, or crudely by using the following formula (220 – your age).

2. Calculate your training heart rate (THR)

THR should be at least 60% of the MHR. Beyond 70% of MHR exercise would be classed as vigorous and at 70-80% you would be in the zone where aerobic conditioning improves the most. So if you are 50 years old the calculation would be:
(220-50)x70% = 133. At that level you would be able to have a conversation with a little bit of puffing.

3. Discover your resting heart rate (RHR)

This is your heart rate when you wake up in the morning before getting out of bed. The average for men is 60-80 beats per minute, and for women 70-90 beats per minute. Athletes tend to be 40-50 beats per minute. The higher your heart rate (RHR), you will notice a drop of one beat per week during the first ten weeks of starting to exercise. You can count it on one side of the Adam's Apple on your neck or on your wrist above the crease on the thumb side.

How Much Exercise Do I Need and How Often?

The minimum is 20 minutes of brisk exercise three times a week. You will need five minutes to warm up and another five minutes for cooling down. If this is the minimum, then five times a week would be better, or a longer session within reason may be better still. A psychiatrist who specialises in stress says the sooner you can take physical action when faced with stress the less the stress will affect you.

Keep smiling. Some people over the age of 60 will walk five miles a day in Britain.

Exercise will keep you fit and healthy, make you feel happier and enhance your creative thinking, and permit meditation; it is also fun. Not least of these advantages is that it will contribute to longer life.

Chapter 7
Look After Your Soul

The Hebrew term for soul is "nephesh" which is the engine of physical life and is mentioned 780 times in the Old Testament. King James uses 28 different words by which to translate the original term, therefore signifies different things depending on the passage in which it occurs. Tanki Tauber defined the soul as the self, "I", that inhabits the body or the life of a person. Without the soul, the body is like a bulb without electricity, a computer without software, a space suit with no astronaut inside. With the introduction of the soul, the body acquires life, sight, hearing, thought and speech.

Every body has a soul and in truth it is not only the human being; every created entity pocesses a 'soul'. Animals, plants, even inanimate objects, every blade of grass and every grain of sand has a soul. Not only life but also existence requires a soul to sustain it - a 'spark of Godliness' that perpetually imbues its object with being and significance. A soul is not just the engine of life. It also embodies the why of a thing's existence, its meaning and purpose. It is a thing's 'inner identity, its raison d'être. Just like the 'soul' of the musical composition is the composer's vision that energizes and gives life to the notes played in a musical composition, the actual notes like the body expressing the vision and feeling of the soul within them. Each soul is the expression of God's intent and vision in creating that particular being.

A person, biological life, mind of a man is characterised by intellectual, creative and emotional characters (Gen. 27:25). If

49

he talks about it as the spirit it is the eternal component of man that is fashioned in the very image of God. (Gen. 1:26), and that can exist apart from the physical body, (Matthew 10:28, Rev 6:9).

The Apostle Paul, writing to the Romans, again connects the body, the mind (soul) and the spirit. He refers to the mind as the soul.

St Paul, looking intently at the Council, said, "Brethren, I have lived my life with a perfectly good conscience before God up to this day." (Acts 23:1 NASB)

Therefore I urge you, brethren, by the mercies of God, to present your bodies a living and holy sacrifice, acceptable to God, which is your spiritual service of worship. And do not be conformed to this world, but be transformed by the renewing of your mind, so that you may prove what the will of God is, that which is good and acceptable and perfect. (Romans 12:1-2 NASB).

The Soul (Greek, "psyche")

Genesis 2:7 states that Man was created as a "living soul." The soul consists of the mind (which includes the conscience), the will and the emotions. The soul and the spirit are mysteriously tied together and make up what the Scriptures call the "heart."

The writer of Proverbs declares, "Watch over your heart with all diligence, for from it flow the springs of life." (Prov. 4:23 NASB). We see here that the "heart" is central to our emotions and will.

But a natural (psuchikos -- soulish) man does not accept the things of the Spirit of God, for they are foolishness to him; and he cannot understand them, because they are spiritually appraised. (1 Cor. 2:14 NASB).

According to the Bible, mankind is distinct from all the rest of creation, including the animals, in that he is made in the image of God. As God is a tripartite -- Father, Son and Holy Spirit -- so man is three parts -- body, soul and spirit. In the most explicit example from Scripture of these divisions, the Apostle Paul writes:

Now may the God of peace Himself sanctify you entirely; and may your spirit and soul and body be preserved complete, without blame at the coming of our Lord Jesus Christ. (1 Thessalonians 5:23 NASB)

Chapter 8
Look After Your Spirit

In the Old Testament spirit is rauch, literally meaning breath, "wind", etc. It is found 378 times in the Hebrew Old Testament. The corresponding Greek term is pnuema, occurring 379 times in the New Testament. Again, the word "spirit" may take on a different sense, depending on its contextual setting. The non-physical being. It is also used to depict the nature of non-material being, e.g. God (the Father). The same applies to the Holy Spirit as to his essence, is spirit Jn 4:24 . Similarly the angels are spirit in nature.

A person's spirit can be used by the way of the figure of speech known as synecdoche (part of the whole).

The spirit of the human being can be defined as the eternal part of the human body, which differentiates him from animals, who only have body and soul. The spirit of the human being has the power to think, create and innovate. All the technology and science that led man to land on the moon and create the technology for gadgets such as television, computers, internet, cars, is only possible for man to achieve. In Christianity they believe the spirit is the part of the human body that will go to heaven when he or she dies. The great God the Creator has created the human being as small Gods to work, discover, innovate and improve our life on earth. To have a balanced life we need to communicate with our creator, whether through meditation or prayer, to get us into a state of peace and serenity. I remember when I was a young doctor there was a clinical trial about heart patients who were having heart surgery. Half of them had prayers before the operation and the other half did not. The result of this trial showed that patients who had prayer before their operation had better results and a more speedy recovery than the ones who had not prayed. Our spirits long to go to heaven where they came from and our bodies long to go to earth where they came from.

Spiritual Healing

Christian View

Healing or cure

If you have a body illness you go to a doctor to treat the disease or cure it.

If you have a spiritual problem some people ignore it. Jesus was like a doctor in the 4 gospels; he cured people's illnesses, the bodily and spiritual illness or the psychological. He cured the blind, the deaf, the paralytic and the possessed of the evil spirit.

Fathers of the church concentrated on the spiritual healing, which is more common than body illnesses. Body blindness people know about, but spiritual blindness many of us do not know about it. St Paul thought he could see well but when he met Jesus he became blind. Jesus wanted to tell him that he had been blind for a long time and would need a miracle. After being baptised he went to Ananias, and got baptised when some scales came out of his eyes and he started to see. He was blind about God and now he could see. If there is a gathering of people, how many people are blind? There may be none or just a few. If you ask about spiritual blindness you will find a lot, including myself.

One of the monks spoke to his spiritual adviser saying, "I want to perform a miracle like Jesus", to which his adviser replied, "If you want to cure a paralysed man there is an easy way to do it. If you find somebody who does not go to church, ask him to go to church so he was paralysed but can walk to the church now. If you find a man who is blind spiritually ask him to read the Bible and learn the praises of God. If you find someone who is deaf spiritually ask him to go to a retreat away from the noises of the world and he will start to hear the word of God. If you want to raise a dead person invite a person who is away from God to church so he will get to know God.

Spiritual healing is more important than bodily healing, as he who will get a bodily illness cured and live for years will eventually die, but if his spirit is cured he will live forever. If you are not cured of a spiritual problem the result will be eternal death.

According to the teaching of Jesus, someone who judges others daily and thinks he is perfect, judging others in his own eyes, mind and thought and words, is very dangerous. Do not judge so you cannot be judged. He said, "Get the specks out of your eyes before judging others." It is a very common spiritual disease and some people ignore it and consider it normal.

Another example is anger during driving, at work or in social life. Jesus said that he who becomes angry against his brother will be judged. Who says to his brother ' You good for nothing' shall be in danger of the council. So we should not be angry; if you are always angry your blood pressure will go up, you could get diabetes, even a brain haemorrhage in extreme cases.

You will go to your doctor for bodily diseases or for checkups, but for anger you ignore it although it is serious and can take you to the council.

There are other spiritual diseases which are not apparent because they are hidden, like bad thoughts, or planning evil things for other people. It could be somebody who had a bad experience in his childhood, e.g. abuse, divorce or violence between his parents, which left him with psychological problems, or a wound so he or she might be anxious, depressed, or frightened of other people.

They may feel there is no peace in their heart and all because of the wounds of their childhood. Spiritual Healing can clear away all these problems and reconcile him with God and the people around him.

Jesus came to cure all our sins. He carried it and bore our pain and lifted them on the cross.

How can we get cured spiritually? With a bodily illness, the most important thing is to make a diagnosis: x-rays, scans, MRI, history, examination and blood tests. The same applies to spiritual healing.

Suppose somebody gets angry very easily, it could be –

1. Love of money
2. Proud of himself
3. Fear of people around him
4. Belittling or undervaluing the self
5. Hating people or a specific person

All of these are symptoms and the origin is Anger; the treatment is different for every symptom in the spiritual world.

Another example, judging other people and their symptoms.

1. Jealousy – he tries to destroy another person to prove he is better than them.
2. Proud of himself
3. Lack of love

Jesus used to treat the cause but not the symptom.

Examples:

The Samaritan woman
The symptom is she went with several men and people judged her. She was a sinner and people did not respect her. On the other hand, when Jesus met her he diagnosed her as needing love and respect. She had been wrongly brought up and had low self-esteem. According to the judgement of others she should be stoned, but when Jesus met her and talked to her she thought he was a prophet, then realised he was the Messiah. She invited people to see him and when they met him they believed, not because of the Samaritan woman but because they had seen Him and talked to Him.

The woman who was "caught in the act"
People judged her and called her an adulterer but Jesus diagnosed her as depressed, a badly treated woman in a sinful society. He treated her nicely and wrote the sins of the people around her on earth, and said to them "he who has no sin should stone her" but they all went away. Then he looked towards her and said, "nobody had judged you, go and do not sin again", and she was cured. If people had stoned her she would not have been cured.

The bleeding woman who touched the hem of Jesus's garment
She was legally unclean. She was suffering and anaemic, emaciated and had been bleeding for 12 years. The people said she was unclean and should not touch anyone. She felt that she

was not accepted by God. She thought if she could steal a touch of Jesus, the bleeding would stop and if she went home the feeling of guilt would not go as she considered herself an unclean woman. When she did touch Jesus she was sure she had made him unclean. Although everyone was touching him, this time he stopped and asked "Who touched me?" because power had come out of him. So she came forward and told him her story. She said she had been bleeding for 12 years and was desperate to be cured and so she had touched his garments. She asked why he did not get angry with her. He said nobody has judged you "Woman, your faith has healed you, go in peace". She went home cured of her bodily illness (the bleeding) but more importantly from her spiritual illness, the feeling of guilt that she was unclean, the feeling of belittling herself, the feeling that everyone around her thought she was unclean.

The prodigal son
He took his share of money (his inheritance) whilst his father was still alive, although it is normally taken after the death of parents. On this occasion, he had taken his money before the death of his father because he was an ungrateful, inconsiderate person. He eventually lost all the money, having spent it on his pleasures, only to find himself being unable to feed himself and lusted to eat some of the pigs' food. Then he realised that the servants of his father were eating better food than him. He thought he would go back to his father and ask if he could be a servant in his house. For the father to accept him is not a problem. But there are more spiritual problems; the feeling of guilt that he lost all his father's money, disgracing his father by his bad reputation, destroying his father's reputation by treating him as though he were dead whilst he was still alive. But the loving father, when he heard that his son was coming back, ran towards him, cuddled him with joy, gave him a nice suit and held a big reception for him. He wanted to forgive him and cure him of all the guilt he was feeling and did not ask his son about

his loss, mismanagement or disgraceful behaviour. He wanted to cure him from all the guilt he was suffering and start a new page with him. He said, "My son was dead and now he is alive"; it was as if he did not do anything wrong.

Spiritual Healing needs the following:

I.   The right diagnosis. The Bible and the church set rules that there are deputy doctors who are the priests who can diagnose your spiritual problems and give you a solution. In the Old Testament the priest can judge when a leper can go back into the community after he is cured. Nowadays, if someone complains that he is always judging people and feeling angry, a priest will diagnose his problem whether he is proud of himself, loves or worships money, undermines himself or hates other people. He will give him advice to sort out his problems. The only people Jesus was hard on were the Pharisees and scribes, who were bad teachers and hypocrites who were more concerned about politics and themselves than religion.

II. Go and see a spiritual healer. In normal medicine when a patient goes to his own doctor with too many symptoms the doctor will try to diagnose the main problem or disease that is causing all the symptoms. The same applies to spiritual healing. St John summarised the spiritual diseases into three major parts:

a] Lust of the Flesh
b] Lust of the Eyes
c] Living in a Luxurious and Pompous Manner

So the three main spiritual diseases are self love, love of money/worshipping money and lust of the body. If somebody is always irritable, cannot tolerate any criticism and hates other people, his main problem is that he loves himself and is egotistical.

III. St Anthony used to say if you have a spiritual problem, e.g. anger or swearing, read St James 3 and learn to verses by heart.

1 My brethren, be not many masters, knowing that we shall receive the greater condemnation.

2 For in many things we offend all. If any man offend not in word, the same is a perfect man, and able also to bridle the whole body.

3 Behold, we put bits in the horses' mouths, that they may obey us; and we turn about their whole body.

4 Behold also the ships, which though they be so great, and are driven of fierce winds, yet are they turned about with a very small helm, whithersoever the governor listeth.

5 Even so the tongue is a little member, and boasteth great things. Behold, how great a matter a little fire kindleth!

6 And the tongue is a fire, a world of iniquity: so is the tongue among our members, that it defileth the whole body, and setteth on fire the course of nature; and it is set on fire of hell.

7 For every kind of beasts, and of birds, and of serpents, and of things in the sea, is tamed, and hath been tamed of mankind:

8 But the tongue can no man tame; it is an unruly evil, full of deadly poison.

9 Therewith bless we God, even the Father; and therewith curse we men, which are made after the similitude of God.

10 Out of the same mouth proceedeth blessing and cursing. My brethren, these things ought not so to be.

11 Doth a fountain send forth at the same place sweet water and bitter?

12 Can the fig tree, my brethren, bear olive berries? either a vine, figs? so can no fountain both yield salt water and fresh.

13 Who is a wise man and endued with knowledge among you? let him shew out of a good conversation his works with meekness of wisdom.

14 But if ye have bitter envying and strife in your hearts, glory not, and lie not against the truth.

15 This wisdom descendeth not from above, but is earthly, sensual, devilish.

16 For where envying and strife is, there is confusion and every evil work.

17 But the wisdom that is from above is first pure, then peaceable, gentle, and easy to be intreated, full of mercy and good fruits, without partiality, and without hypocrisy.

18 And the fruit of righteousness is sown in peace of them that make peace.

By remembering it and rehearsing the words you will reduce your anger and swearing.

IV. Meeting with Jesus Himself

All of us have iniquities, have old spiritual wounds, have our old guilts and bad experiences. But when we come close to Jesus these problems will dissolve. He will carry all our iniquities and give us the forgiveness and comfort of our spirit and can heal all our wounds.

Church Healing

Amputation or Prayer?
Word quickly began to spread of the healing miracles that were taking place among the worker in the Muqattam churches and people started to bring relatives and friends from outside their area to receive prayer for healing. Caroline, a girl from Heliopolis or "New Cairo", was suffering from a tumour in her upper tibia (part of the shin bone just below the knee). The doctors who had examined her in June 1991 found this to be a malignant tumour called Ewing's Sarcoma. Caroline was only six years old but was suffering from a rare and fatal condition. The only treatment for this was amputation in view of the advanced stage to which the tumour had developed. This had been the only recommendation she was given, even after having travelled to France for specialist investigations; the doctors in Egypt also agreed. Whilst she was awaiting amputation, she underwent radiotherapy and chemotherapy, which resulted in complete hair loss.

However, Caroline's parents had faith in God and were sure He could do something to save her leg. They visited the Coptic monastery of Abu Seifein in Old Cairo, the same site that was rebuilt in the time of Patriarch Abraam. There they were advised to go and see Father Simaan in Muqattam. Having heard about the miracle of the mountain moving helped to strengthen their faith in God and were sure he could intervene in the present just as he had done in the past. They took Caroline to Muqattam where, through the ministry, she developed a personal relationship with God. On 21 August 1994 Father Simaan prayed that she would be healed in the name of Christ. He then told the doctors to stop the radiotherapy and chemotherapy treatment, trusting that Caroline had been healed.

Caroline's parents confirmed in faith and agreed that they did not want the amputation to be carried out. This is not a decision that can be taken lightly as Ewing's Sarcoma typically spreads from the leg to the liver and then the brain, inevitably resulting in death within approximately six months.

But Caroline is today a healthy girl, living in her family's home in Heliopolis "New Cairo".

World Vision Award

By now, Father Simaan had been administering at Muqattam for twenty years. Recognition for his ministry at Muqattam in all its various forms came the year after Caroline's healing in 1995. The Bible Society of Egypt recommended Father Simaan for a special presentation in recognition of his outstanding example in spiritual leadership. The recommendation led to the decision of World Vision International to present Father Simaan with the Robert Pierce Award, the purpose of which is "to provide recognition for those who have contributed in a significant way to the Kingdom of God".

Bruce McConchie, Regional Director of World Vision in the Middle East, came and observed the church's ministry for himself. He described the atmosphere in the Muqattam Mountain site on the night of the presentation: The strains of "He is Lord" rose from the cave as we strode in the Mokattam Coptic Orthodox Church, on the outskirts of Cairo. As the auditorium came into view, the vastness was breathtaking. A huge arc of upward sloping terraces and seats to a charcoal grey crescent at the top where the cave opened to the sky and a single star. Ten thousand people could be seated in this place. The band, choir and congregation could now be seen and heard in one great crescendo of praise to the living Lord and Saviour. We were deep inside the Mokattam Mountain as Father Simon Ibrahim gently guided me into the front rows of the auditorium. The worship continued. Time stood still as I reflected on what I had seen and heard during the previous hours. It had been a non-stop affirmation of transformational development in all its variety and potential. The power of God was inescapable. The impact was evident in the thousands of people seated up to the sky behind me......

Father Simaan received the award in the presence of his congregation, his family and invited guests. It must have been a very proud moment for his wife, Su'aad, who had supported him so faithfully in his ministry. She had managed to hold down the post of General Secretary of a company, while being active in church work and bringing up their two children, Albeer and Mary. These children were now married and were in attendance at the presentation. Albeer had risen to become a company director, and Mary helped to supervise the running of the Patmos Hospital with her husband, Dr Samweel.

Coptic priests representing the Bishop of Shubra El-Kheima diocese (who was abroad) attended the presentation of the award, along with the Director of the Egyptian Bible Society, Ramez Atallah (who had become interested in the ministry at Muqattam for many years). The Reverend Jim Doust was there to represent the Anglican Cathedral in Cairo.

Father Simaan was grateful for the recognition, and this motivated him to pray, "Create in me a clean heart, O God, and put a new and right spirit within me." (Psalms 51.10 RSV). He asked all those present to pray that he would continue to be strengthened and encouraged by the Lord. "Places like Muqattam", he said, "do not satisfy the hearts of men. Only God satisfies the hearts of men. Therefore, you can say, 'I live, yet not I, Christ lives in me!'"

Transformed Lives
The thousands of people who had attended left the auditorium with this challenge ringing in their ears and – he hoped – resonating in their hearts. The gospel continued to make a huge impact on people's lives. The goodness of God continued to be seen in the ministry of the church, the hospital, the kindergarten and lower primary school. His abundant provision was seen in vocational training activities and encouragement for small businesses. Lives continued to be transformed by these projects. A good example of this was Jehan, a girl from a very poor family, who had graduated from the church school. She joined the Vocational Training Workshop and became skilled in making attractive handicrafts from recycled cloth. Her work helped immensely in raising the standard of living for her family. Jehan became one of the first Zaballeen girls to travel. She represented the workshop abroad at international conferences concerned with recycling. The workshop and Jehan's projects to kick-start small businesses were playing an initial and important role in a population living in and around the mountain that had now reached a total of 40,000 people.

The Impossible Dilemma
Miracles of healing continued to occur. For example, there was an urgent crisis to be faced regarding a young couple, Nahid and her husband, Mahir. Nahid noticed that she was losing weight rapidly. When her weight dropped from 11 stone to 7½ stone she went to see a doctor, who immediately took some blood tests. Nahid was also suffering from terrible headaches.

She was prescribed antibiotics, but before long the doctor referred her to Ein Shams Hospital. After undergoing the usual x-rays Mahir, her husband, was informed by the consultant that Nahid needed a brain scan. As the equipment for this was not available at his hospital Nahid was taken to a specialist centre. When they went back to their consultant he told Mahir that his wife's condition was extremely serious. He said that she had a swelling on the outer layer of the brain, known as an extradural haematoma. This external symptom was linked to an internal problem in the brain. There was a major artery in the brain that had aneurism – a condition that causes sudden dilatation or haemorrhaging of the wall of the blood vessel, eventually causing a haemorrhage in the brain. It was possible that this rupture would occur within 72 hours.

Doctors also told Nahid that they would have to perform open heart surgery as tests had shown that she was suffering from cardiomyopathy – a condition affecting the muscles of the heart which, in some cases, can result in a heart attack. Shortly after being given this diagnosis Nahid lost consciousness and Mahir found himself faced with an impossible dilemma. The doctors had said that in order to save Nahid they would have to operate on both her heart and her brain; one operation without the other would be no good. It was not good enough to operate only on the valves in the heart that were malfunctioning , as if they did not deal with the dilated artery in the brain, and the brain would inevitably haemorrhage within 72 hours. Mahir knew that to agree to this double operation was a huge responsibility. The doctors had told him that the risk of something going wrong during such an operation was high and the outcome doubtful in the extreme. Even if the surgery succeeded, Nahid could be left paralysed in both legs. The area in the brain that the surgeons could safely work on was no more than 2.5 sq. cm in area.

Mahir told the doctors that both he and Nahid had a Christian Faith: that if this was impossible for human beings, it could be possible for God. The doctors had not considered this and were not entirely convinced, but they agreed to move Nahid from intensive care to a cardiac ward.

When Mahir called Father Simaan to come and see him, the first thing the Father asked him was, "Do YOU pray or not?" Mahir replied, "I used to pray, but I don't these days".

"Why don't you pray?"

"After I got married I just stopped praying," he confessed.

"Do you have faith or not?"

"I have faith that God will heal her."

Father Simaan had visited while Nahid was unconscious. The heart monitoring equipment was removed and Father Simaan put his hand on her face, making a cross upon it. He then brought a cup of water, prayed over it, and put it to one side. Then he prayed for her. Nahid appeared to be asleep. Father Simaan went and got the water and poured it on her face three times. "After that, our Lord was glorified and the miracle took place," said Mahir. Nahid regained consciousness. Father Simaan spoke to Nahid: "As Christ said, 'Pick up your bed and walk', I say to you, pick up your bed and walk."

He then told her to go home.

Nahid had been used to having four injections every hour, and another injection every four hours. Whilst in hospital she had been given numerous injections of antibiotics and had responded to none of them. But now Father Simaan was telling her to leave the hypodermics behind and go home! In the most natural way she got up and with Mahir's help, packed her belongings and went home.

This happened on Friday, 9 August 1996. Father Simaan had arrived at noon, they went home at 1.00pm. The Surgeon had informed Mahir that he needed one day to prepare for the operation. As the hospital only performed operations on Saturday, Sunday and Monday, it meant they had to make a decision by Friday or Saturday at the latest. By 1.15pm on Friday, Mahir and Nahid had made their decision – there would be no operation.

They telephoned the doctor from home saying that Nahid had been healed by faith. The doctors were not convinced and assumed they must be very ignorant people. How could Nahid have possibly discharged herself when x-rays clearly showed that she had an aneurism in her brain, in addition to which she needed new valves in her heart. But that is exactly what Nahid had done! The threatened haemorrhage never took place, and Nahid made a full recovery.

She gave her testimony to this at Muqattam on 9 September, with her husband, Mahir, and small son. Since Nahid had been unconscious for much of the time, Mahir had to fill in many aspects of the trials they had been through. She had not known about the life-threatening aneurism in her brain, but was now completely free of all symptoms, even the severe headaches suffered in the beginning.

Such testimonies have shown people who have heard them that trials do not have to lead to despair. "Nothing is impossible with God." (Luke 1.37). The believers at Muqattam saw that, by turning a problem into prayer, God could make them "more than conquerors" (Romans 8.37) over everything. These testimonies also affected their view of death. In the Western World people are afraid to talk of death. When someone famous dies suddenly (like Princess Diana) it sends shockwaves around the country, although in ordinary families people will have small, private funerals. By contrast, people in the East drop everything when someone they are acquainted with dies. Men will leave their place of work and women dress in black to go and comfort a bereaved family. Death in Egypt has a higher profile and people will display great, almost uncontrollable emotion at public funerals. The believers at Muqattam began to sense that bodily death did not have to be seen through floods of tears, loss and anguish, but could be understood as the process of being transferred from one state of existence to another. A grey-haired priest who was present at Nahid's public testimony reminded listeners of how Jesus said of the daughter of Jairus, the synagogue ruler, "The child is not dead, but asleep." (Mark 5.39). Then he said to her, "Little girl......arise." (verse 41) just as if He were waking her from a sleep. Sleep here means bodily death. It is sin that is really death.

If we do not hear God's voice calling us in this life, we will hear it on the day of judgement. The miracle God really wants to do is the miracle of raising us from the death of Sin.

If you are ill in Egypt, you can pay a huge sum of money for the services of a well-known surgeon. But many people, like Nahid and Mahir, can testify that God was able to raise them up not just from their sick bed but from death itself, freely and without charge. To them this is a sign of something infinitely greater. To trust in the blood of Christ is to be truly raised, raised not merely from the death of the body, but of the soul.

Out of the Pit
On 16 October 1996 a young doctor gave a testimony at a meeting in Muqattam. He explained how his preoccupation

with healing the body for a time led him away from the Lord. But God intervened, and turned his priorities upside down.

"I was suffering from three slipped discs in the lower part of my back. A doctor told me to rest. After five weeks he told me I should be able to return to my normal everyday life. What was my everyday life like? I had known the Lord for about fifteen years, having had experience of meeting him personally. Yet after starting work I found very little time for him. I told myself that this was not the same as being at school or university; I was now in the world of work, which was completely different. There was no time for ministry. Anyway, I assured myself, medicine is a kind of ministry, and this helped ease my conscience.

There came a time when I suffered three slipped discs and for the five weeks I was advised to rest by the doctor I felt unable to get out of bed except to go to the toilet. At the end of that time I managed to sit in a chair, but after only five minutes of sitting I felt a sharp pain in my back that transmitted down one leg. I mentioned this to the doctor and said I was now beginning to feel pain down my right side as well as the left. The doctor was a well-known specialist in bone diseases and said, "You can do one of two things, you can either take to your bed and stay there for a few months, or if you are a man who earns a thousand dollars a day, I can do an operation tomorrow. It will not cure the problem immediately but could speed up the recovery time." His words did not encourage me and I found I couldn't get out of bed, and became depressed. My brother was going to visit a priest so I asked him, "Tell the priest that I am ill." When the priest arrived I asked him two questions, but they were not about healing. Although I was a believer, the issue of healing was not what was occupying my thoughts. What I wanted to know was, "Does God want to say something to me through this illness?" and secondly, "Where was the wisdom of

God in leaving me unable to work and support my family?"

Father Simaan came and I asked him, "Is there anything you want to say about my illness?", to which he replied "No." So I asked, "Is my illness something to do with my spiritual condition?"

"I don't know" he replied, but added "You should ask God and he will tell you."

Then he asked a question of his own saying, "Do you believe that Jesus Christ heals you?"

Matthew prayed, quoting two Bible verses. Then he commanded, "Get up," and I got up.

"Move your head." I moved it.

"Now walk to the other end of the flat." I walked.

"Come back." I came back.

Finally, he said, "Congratulations, God has cured you!" I went over and kissed him (a culturally normal thing for men to do in the Middle East, particularly as a mark of respect for a priest). I saw him to the door, where I hesitated and asked cautiously, "Can I move about now?"

"Yes, you can even run and jump," he replied.

"Run and jump." I felt exhilarated. I proceeded to shave off my beard, got myself dressed and went to find my wife. I also wanted to go and greet my father and brother. I spent two hours just bumping up and down in a car seat.

I was taught as part of my medical training that if you put a lot of weight on one disc it will transmit pressure to the next, and if a good deal of pressure is put on the spinal cord (e.g. jolting up and down) with the condition that I had, it could lead to paralysis of the leg. I, therefore, felt that people seeing me do this would try and stop me from moving around. I knew that even when I found the courage to tell people I had been healed, they would say, "Even so, you must take it easy and don't do this or that." However, I was determined not to give in to any such pressure.

This determination was put to the test when I began to feel again, on and off. I saw this as a challenge and read through the Gospel of Matthew, highlighting in colour all the statements relating to healing. Armed with these verses, I felt fully equipped to fight a spiritual battle. This battle went on for four days as I insisted, no matter what temptation the devil may try to make me believe otherwise, that God had healed me. At the end of this time the pain finally subsided. For the past four months I have been living a very normal life without any recurrence of the illness.

Remarkable as it may seem, this healing was not just God touching my body. Much more powerful than the physical healing was the fact that God gave me joy in my life! This joy meant more to me than anything else and once again I became open to ministry. I offered everything back to the Lord, the hospital, my work, my leisure time. I said to Him, "Take my hand and lead me anywhere you want, anywhere at all. All that matters to me is that I should be in your kingdom."

I have seen myself a lot of miracles in Egypt, by God or saints interceding to God, or by priests or monks in the monasteries who were having a special gift of healing from God. I was still there when St Mary appeared in Zaitoun in April 1968 and her apparition continued for more than a year, which is unique in the world. A lot of miracles happened when they visited her. People were cured, and doctors could not explain it except as a miracle.

Other religions have their own views and believe in spiritual healing. Some believe in energy and they claim they can cure or heal some illnesses by balancing the energy of the body. Others have special prayers or rituals to cure or heal. Also there are some spiritual healers who are possessed by an evil spirit.

Can it harm?
The short answer is yes, if you choose a wrong healer, as some of them are after fame and fortune and of lower spiritual level. they are most likely targeted by ghosts. Higher level ghosts use these defects and attachments in the spiritual healer to affect and possess them. The possession is usually insidious and the healer wouldn't have the faintest idea that he is controlled by a ghost, or sometimes by more than one ghost. Hence it goes unnoticed. Once they have possessed the healer, they initially alleviate the symptoms of the persons treated by the healer through their spiritual strength to gain their faith but also infuse black energy into the person who is treated.

If the healer does not have an advanced sixth sense he may not be able to discern the difference between positive and negative in the spiritual world. Hence, while the healer may think that he is channeling energy from spirit guides he is actually healing with black energy of ghosts posing as spirit guides. So even though the initial may be cured to gain the patient's faith, the long-term effect is damaging.

It is a big subject and you have to choose somebody who has experience and evidence of what he does.

Dr Jean Huston wrote about the universe and your potential power to improve life in this world whatever is your believes.

Three Keys to Unlocking Your Quantum Power - Evolving Wisdom

You are a universe in quantum powers (QP)

We live in a universe and the universe lives in us.

- living a life without limitation
- how to reveal the power of inner goodness and goodness
- new perception of the universe
- people are frustrated because they think about themselves

Dream you have the capacity to live a new life and a new reality.

Live in old beliefs, fire in the belly, creative, bigger vision, you become a magnificent human.

QP unlocking physical ventures, regenesis

You will find –
- how to unlock the QP. Transformation, symptoms, connections, desires, lack of reality.
- Nature of reality We live in a cave, live in a shadow, transform, education, awareness, more capacity if you think the universe lives in them when we live in the shadow.
- Our creative perception, imagining, creative.

1. True Nature of Reality living in a cave

Understanding the immortality, tremors treasure of Buda. How to bring the Tremors to the quantum field.

2. Living New Story Higher Order of Manifestation

True nature of reality to live new life, new storage, how to get rid of waste -> 2m/year remarkable higher operating system.

3. Living in the Light of Expectation

True inner energy. You discover you are the light of quantum power, we have potential.

Who you are -> part of universe imagine a field inside you.
        Power to orchestrate the time.
        Improve skill, higher skills of relativity.

Chapter 7
Have a Healthy Lifestyle

The term "lifestyle" can denote the interests, opinions, or behavioural orientations of an individual, group or culture.

Individual Identity. Not all aspects of lifestyle are voluntary. Surrounding social and technical systems can constrain the lifestyle available to the individual and the symbols an individual is able to project to others and the self.

Health. An individual's health depends a lot on their lifestyle. Maintaining physical, mental, spiritual health is crucial to an individual's longevity. The more time spent on hygiene, physical fitness, diet regulations, meditation or prayer, the healthier lifestyle they will enjoy. Parents are the first teachers for every child. Everything a parent does will very likely transfer to their children through a natural learning process.

One of the most important things is the food we eat. If your weight is not ideal and you want to lose weight, you might think of taking tablets or capsules, maybe starve yourself or start to do more exercise, but these may not work. Many nutritionists believe that you can lose weight by eating a balanced diet and avoiding certain foods and getting the right amount of exercise. There are five foods you should not eat if you wish to lose weight:

1. Concentrated fruit juice
2. Margarine
3. Whole grain bread

4. Soya processed food or milk
5. Corn, especially genetically modified crops

Some people will try taking pills, eating small "cardboard" meals only fit for a small child, or go on a fat-free diet, but when they go back to normal food they find they begin to gain weight and are back to square one.

Watching what you eat and give up eating the previously mentioned food can reduce the belly fat and the whole body fat. Losing weight will make you happier, give you more energy, improve your skin and will prevent aches and pains.

Concentrated Fruit Juice
They remove the fibre which contains nutritious elements and you are left with a bit of juice to which sugar is added, so you are in effect drinking mainly sugary water. If you start your day with a glass of concentrated orange juice the sugar will put the body into a fat storage mode. When blood sugar level is high the body will produce more insulin and the excess sugar is stored as fat. The same applies to most processed food.

Margarine
Margarine is a trans-fat contained in many types of food, e.g. cookies, doughnuts, cakes and fries which contain hydrogenated oil. This is why butter is much better than margarine and unsaturated fat found in almonds, vegetables, fish and olive oil. Saturated fat is found in beef, pizza, ice-cream. Saturated and unsaturated fat in the right combination and quantity will work together to prevent heart attacks and strokes. The right ratio of low carbohydrates and high carbohydrates (sugar) to protein will promote the body to a "burning fat" mode.

Cortisol is a hormone which is produced by the suprarenal gland. When you are in a stressful situation the body produces cortisol and adrenaline to get out of trouble. When you undergo mental stress the body produces also cortisol as it does not differentiate between physical and mental stress.

Whole Wheat Bread
There are 128 calories in one slice of whole wheat bread, and more than 250 calories in a slice of home-made bread. The commercial one contains approximately 80 calories, which is almost similar to white bread (70 calories a slice). Carbohydrates raise the blood sugar. The glycaemic index is broken down into;
low (< 55)
medium (56-69)
high (70-100)

The goal is to get most of your carbohydrates from food rated low to medium on the glycaemic index. Whole grain bread contains three parts of the grain, the germ, the bran and endosperm. The germ and bran contain most of the nutrients (minerals, fibre, essential fats and phyto nutrients).

In the USA and Canada the manufacturers of bread sometimes add only part of the bran and germ and add colouring by adding blackstrip molasses to make the bread look brown.

Therefore, when you are buying bread you should:
- Check the ingredients, whole or whole grain before the name of the grain (whole grain contains more fibre).
- Check the glycaemic index and if not written on the product, you can contact the manufacturer.
- Look at the list of ingredients rather than the colour, to select whole grain food. Eating the right type of bread can help lower the risk of cardiovascular disease, Type II diabetes and obesity. Different companies use different ingredients, so check how many calories per slice are in their particular bread.

Processed Soya Food or Milk

Such foods (and milk) supply energy and put your body into fat storing mode, with no nutrients. Your body produces a hormone known as Ghrelin, so you are able to eat food which is metabolised and gives you the right nutrients, which will make a difference.

Genetically Modified Maize or Corn

This process is banned in Germany, France, Italy and Poland. It is used to fatten livestock, but harmful chemicals are added to it which increases obesity and diabetes.

Primal Blueprint Style of Living

It is about getting the greatest health and fitness benefits that you can with the least amount of suffering, pain or sacrifice.

You can change a large percentage of the food that occupies your kitchen and fridge, and the shift will improve your metabolism and health. You do not need much exercise and many people say you need just 20 minutes of brisk walking every day to keep fit. Blueprint philosophy offers tremendous flexibility for personal preference. You can be sure that you can walk your talk, but you say, I am no ascetic or tightly wound fitness freak.

Three weeks transformation that will last the rest of your life

To live a primal life by eating and exercising primally you will change from a sugar-dependent, fat storing organism that constantly battles hunger, illness and depression and weight gain, into a fat-burning beast who burns stored body fat day and night. You will balance the hormones that were thrown out of balance by hectic modern life. You will have an elevated immune system with high energy levels throughout the day, even when resting.

Eating primally will normalise your insulin levels and reprograme your genes to burn stored body fat for energy. You can go to Marksdailyapple.com to see the success stories.

Do we need carbohydrates?

We get energy from carbohydrates, protein and fat. Food, exercise and lifestyle behaviour that sustained evolution have shaped and moulded the modern genome (complete collection of genetic material). So modelling the lifestyle of our hunter/gatherer ancestors will provide the ingredients to complete our personal recipe for a lean, strong, fit, healthy and happy human being.

If survival is for the fittest and they are able to survive and reproduce in very harsh environmental circumstances, that has refined and perfected the human genetic recipe. Those who did not adapt died out; those lazy, slow, stupid, weak genetic attributes were lost forever. If we call our ancestors a Grok (Primal human role model) the recipe and ingredients to maximise our health and wellbeing are right in front of us, but modern humans seem to disrespect and disregard the profound legacy of our ancestors. It is hard to believe that we are the same inside as the lion-clothed Gork who lived 10,000 years ago. They had no, or little, heart disease, cancer, diabetes or auto-immune diseases. They lived on meat, fish, poultry, insects, eggs, nuts, plants, and fruits, and engaged in a variety of physical exercise. Humans today have switched to eating brand new agricultural foods (wheat, barley, peas, lentils were among the first cultivated crops). On the other hand, the initial generation of predominantly grain-based eaters, such as Egyptians 7,000 years ago, were shorter, less muscular and had a lower bone density than their predecessors. This detrimental effect was due to gene adaptation to new foods. Thousands of years later, with all the recent technology, scientific and medical advancement and discoveries, we are almost in the same situation today and our genes have adapted to this. We are expected to eat high fat dietary food and when we eat agricultural food our bodies consider most of them poisonous because our guts have not adapted. Our genes see an over-abundance of sugar as toxic and take dramatic steps to save us. It sees our lack of exercise, sleep, and sunlight as problematic because we have adapted to being indoors, largely sedentary and blasted with excess artificial light. If we look at the population of the most developed, affluent countries, they have become the fattest, least fit people in the history of mankind. Grok enjoyed a truly healthy lifestyle, whether living to the age of 30, 50 or 70 years.

In contrast, in Western nations, living over the age of eighty is tainted by a deplorable decline in health. Today's exploding population generates tremendous genetic diversity and each of us responds to environmental signals – food, workouts, sleep and sun exposure – that direct our own unique, ideal genetic expression. The good news is that to be healthy you don't have to do extreme training or resort to restrictive/obsessive dietary habits, nor adopt joyless/Spartan daily regimes. The right amount and quality of food, exercise, meditation and sleep can change your life. Our ancestors ate little carbohydrates. If you eat excess carbohydrates you will over-stress your insulin response system and become insulin resistant. This could mean big trouble for you as your body will store your excess carbohydrates as glycogen and fat and if not efficiently processed (burnt, stored as glycogen or as fat) it will damage protein molecules through a process called "glycolism." This will lead to various disease problems associated with obesity and Type II diabetes, and systemic inflammation. There is no requirement to dietary carbohydrates in human nutrition. Your body can manufacture glucose on demand, which is essential for your brain, from proteins and fat to keep you focused and energetic. This process is called "gluconeogencis". Your brain can work more efficiently with Ketones than with glucose, probably because of our ancestors' ability to access Ketones rather than glucose.

If you eat 50-100g./day of carbohydrate you will lose weight and if you eat100-150g., which can be gained from fruits and vegetables, you will maintain your weight. If you eat 150-300g. you will have insidious weight gain and that will lead to widespread health conditions. And, if you eat more than 300g. that might lead metabolic syndrome, obesity,type 2 Diabetes and other various health problems.

The most important hormone is insulin

Insulin has a profound influence on the body composition. Studies have investigated other hormones (Glucagon, Cortisol, Leptin, Ghrelin, Adrenalin, Nor-adrenalin, PPY, T3, testosterone, human growth hormones, and many more) on hunger, appetite, satiety, inflammation, obesity, diabetes and metabolism, but the most important one was insulin. The more you secrete insulin during your lifetime the shorter time you will live. When you chronically over-produce insulin as a sugar burner and fail to empty muscle glycogen and replenish it with regular exercise, you become insulin resistant. This will lead to various diseases such as atherosclerosis (hardening of the arteries), appetite hormone get thrown out of balance causing you to eat when you should feel satiated, and your body stores any excess sugar as fat. Melatonin and Serotonin cycles get messed up and you can end up feeling grumpy and groggy in the morning, and crave sugar in the evenings. This can also lead to sleep deprivation. When you are able to optimise your insulin production, sex hormones are delivered properly to the target organs, cholesterol assist with energy and hormone production and appetite, sleep and thyroid hormone become balanced. Insulin resistance occurs when muscle and liver cells become desensitised to insulin's storage signals due to excessive production. This will promote obesity, accelerated ageing, atherosclerosis, sleep deprivation and type 2 diabetes.

Your day-to-day health is greatly influenced by the quality of your last meal. Eat just a few low insulin producing meals, and you are likely to experience an improvement in a appetite, energy levels, sleep cycles and other sensations of vitality. The combination of blood glucose spike and insulin triggered glucose crash leads to a physical, mental and emotional lull which is best described as burnout.

As we have seen before, exercise is ineffective in weight management.

Frequent to medium to difficult exercise promotes consumption of additional calories and less general activity in the ensuing hours. This compensation asserts itself that exercise cancels itself out as regards to weight management. Muscles burn minimally more calories than fat at rest, and that is invalidates the influence of fitness on weight management. Our genes need two to five hours a week of low intensity exercise for maximum health benefits, in addition to structured aerobic at 55- 75 per cent of maximum heart rate, as it is critical to move around more during our daily life, avoiding the sedentary life. If you exercise hard above 75 per cent of maximum heart rate, it will increase stress, suppress the immune function, compromise weight- loss efforts and promote burnout.

Sometimes your genes expect you to challenge body by doing short intense workouts that will help build strength, speed and power.

Some people believe that the more time they spend at the gym in an exhausting attempt to build their muscles and get fit, the better results they get. This is not true. The truth is, once you understand that 80 per cent of your body composition is determined by your diet, you will understand that you can get really fit in a short time.

Primal blueprint fitness recommends
Sprint, All out efforts <10 minutes per 7-10 days
Lift heavy things brief intense sessions of full-body functional movements
1-3 times per week for 7-30 minutes.
Move frequently at slow pace
Waking, hiking, cycling, easy cardio 55-75%of maximum heart rate for 2-5 hours per week.

They claim this will promote lifelong functional fitness, and support a lean toned physique by eating primally.

Instead of leading a sedentary, robotic, consistency-obsessed approach to life, favoured by conventional wisdom , feel free to try an intuitive approach to primal exercise.

Ageing
Modern hectic life is contributing to the process of ageing by eating in the blood sugar-burning zone, excess stress levels, poor exercise habits (either chronic or insufficient) and poor lifestyle habits (lack of sufficient sleep, sun and play).

Overly training exercise can suppress the key vitality hormones such as testosterone or human growth hormone, and can compromise immune system to the extent of 6 - 8 attacks of chest infection per year, bowel diseases such as irritable bowel syndrome, bloating and constipation, osteoarthritis, chronic fatigue and ultimately physical and psychological burnout.

Training our genes by eating the right food will promote optimal gene expression that make us look good and be at our best.

Primal Diet Recommendation

Meat and Poultry

Meat, poultry, fish and eggs will provide the bulk of your dietary calories, as these foods are excellent sources of saturated fat and complete protein that support all angles of your health. The best end of spectrum for meat and poultry would start with lean, high omega-3 wild animal brought down by bow and arrow in the Alaskan wilderness. Next would be pastured or 100% grass fed animal raised in your local area. Organic animals have access to the outdoors by law but are typically fed by grains. In many cases they are inferior   to animals raised in pastures eating mostly grass, insects and other element of their diet as this diet will boost omega-3 and other nutrients. These could be found in farmers markets, local butchers and online. Unfortunately the vast majority of animal products offered today are produced by intensive factory farming and they are inferior to organic animals, and they can taste differently.

Eggs

Can be enjoyed in abundance as a centrepiece of a healthy diet. They used to say egg consumption should moderated or (eat the white and not the yolks which is high in cholesterol) which is untrue. Egg yolk is one of the most nutritious foods on earth, full of antioxidants and anti-inflammatory agents and a complete amino acid profile, omega-3 fats, saturated fats,vitamins A, E, K2 and B complex.

Try to eat eggs from grass fed chickens, these are the highest on the spectrum and contain up to 10 times of omega-3s than conventionally raised eggs. Next in spectrum are organic eggs which are better than conventional egg as they are free of objectionable hormones, pesticides and antibiotics and poor sanitary living conditions.

Fish

Fish offer excellent nutritional value from complete protein, B complex vitamins, selenium, vitamin D, vitamin E, zinc, iron, magnesium, phosphorus, antioxidants and other nutrients.

Oily, cold water fish from remote, pollution free waters are some of the most nutrient-rich foods on earth. No other food even comes close to the abundant omega-3 levels in wild caught sustainable salmon, sardines, herring, mackerel and anchovies. Fish online can tell you more about how to choose your healthier fish.

Commercially bought fish at the top food chains could contain more mercury, which is toxic to humans when present at certain detectable levels e.g. (tuna, sword fish and sharks, etc)

Perhaps you should avoid most of the farmed fish as they contain toxic chemicals e.g. dioxins dieldrin, toxaphene and other insecticides in addition they give them antibiotics.

If you are going to eat farmed fish you should insist on buying it from domestic   sources which contains less toxins, but not from China.

Vegetables

Vegetables offer excellent antioxidant, micronutrient and anti-inflammatory properties and should form the bulk of your diet relating to the portion size. Adjust your mentality to make veggies a centrepiece of your meals and snacks, get comfortable with consuming larger quantities than the typical western diet traditions call for. Be confident that it takes a heap of veggies to even come close to maxing out you carbohydrate 'budget' for the day.

Try to buy locally grown veggies for freshness.

You can enjoy a bowl of freshly picked garden tomatoes, bag of cooked spinach or head of broccoli for lunch one day.

Different colours of vegetables have specific health benefits: reds are believed to help prevent prostate cancer, greens contribute to anti-ageing and vision, yellow and orange aid immune support and digestion and so on. Concentrate on the idea that abundance of vegetable consumption will promote your general health, and they taste great.

Some of the vegetables with the highest anti oxidant values: beetroot, broccoli, Brussels sprouts, carrots, cauliflower, aubergines, garlic, kale, onion, peas, red peppers, spinach, swiss chard and yellow squash.

Fruits
Fruits are excellent sources of vitamins, fibre, minerals, phenols (anti-oxidant, anti-inflammatory agents) anti-oxidants and other micronutrients, some moderation is warranted for few reasons. The first one - modern cultivation and chemical treatments have resulted in bigger fruits, brightly coloured, uniformly shaped and extra sweet with much less micronutrients than the small, varied, highly fibrous, deep coloured, less sugary and less insulin-stimulating that Grok foraged for.

The second reason is that overly sweet fruits are available all the year around.

The third reason
The fructose which is the predominant carbohydrate form in the fruits can cause significant metabolic problems when consumed in excess even though it generates of less of an immediate insulin spike than other forms of carbohydrate consumption. This is particularly true when fruits are consumed with the excessively high carbohydrate western diet.

Fructose is converted to glucose in the liver but also to triglycerides (fat).

If you ingest excess fructose and your glycogen storage is full, the fructose will convert to triglyceride and be pumped into the blood stream. High triglyceride will interfere with the function of satiety hormone leptin causing you to want to overeat rather than to rely on the body stored fat for energy. Perhaps one third of the population are fructose intolerant to some degree, which is manifested as flatulence.cramps, bloating, irritable bowel syndrome and diarrhoea. Excess fructose can make you fat.

Eat fruits which are local, organic, in season; avoid fruits which are sprayed with pesticides without washing them e.g.berries, apricot, cherries, apples.

You can grow your own fruits or hit the farmers market.

You perhaps have noticed that I have not mentioned carbohydrate as they think that all what require is 100 mg/day and can easily be gained from vegetables and fruits.

[To summarise eating primal diet will train your genes to keep you happy, healthy, energetic, in a fat burning mode rather than fat storing mode. This is one of the many life styles you can follow specially if you wish to keep your weight under control.